"The 'mommy' of all postpartum classes."

New York Times, Women's Health, 6/22/97

. . . . .

"Ms. Trindade, doubly experienced as a mother and trainer, has crafted a program that deals with the physical changes of starting life with a new baby."

Alan Morris, M.D., F.A.C.O.G.

. . . . .

"My mood was up, my worries seemed less, I felt energized and more ready for the rest of the day. My muscles got stronger, and I had fewer aches. My body shape is also changing for the first time in my life."

Janice L. Gelfand, M.D.

. . . . .

"I lost forty-six pounds in seven months, and I am getting a new and slimmer shape, which I didn't have before my baby!"

Kimberly Ajavananda, new mom

. . . . .

"If you do only one thing as a new mother, do Strollercize."

Lisa Larson, new mom

. . . . .

"Strollercize is a must for any new mom."

Claudia Pinto, new mom

. . . . .

"Strollercize was just what the doctor ordered after two pregnancies."

Gina Sisti, new mom

. . . . .

"My greatest fear during pregnancy was losing the forty-five pounds I'd gained. After Strollercizing, I'm several pounds below my prepregnancy weight."

Terry Voltaggio, new mom and investment banker

. . . . .

"Strollercize has really helped me make the transition from professional to mom. It's a great way to lose weight, get fit, and do it all with my baby. Can't say enough good things about it."

Ellyssa Weldon, new mom and T.V. producer

Strollercize®
The Workout for New Mothers

ELIZABETH TRINDADE

and VICTORIA SHAW, Ph.D.

THREE RIVERS PRESS • NEW YORK

Before beginning any new exercise program, including the exercise routine discussed in this book, consult with your physician to make sure it is appropriate for each individual's situation. This program is designed for an individual to perform, not as a group class. The reader should follow all of the instructions carefully and be aware there are always risks in exercising, let alone in a fitness program with a stroller.

Published by Three Rivers Press, New York, New York.
Member of the Crown Publishing Group.

Random House, Inc. New York, Toronto, London, Sydney, Auckland
www.randomhouse.com

THREE RIVERS PRESS is a registered trademark and the
Three Rivers Press colophon is a trademark of Random House, Inc.

Printed in the United States of America

Strollercize® is a registered trademark of Strollercize, Inc., New York City.

Design by Helene Berinsky

Library of Congress Cataloging-in-Publication Data
Trindade, Elizabeth.
Strollercize : the workout for new mothers /
Elizabeth Trindade and Victoria Shaw.
1. Postnatal care.   2. Exercise for women.   3. Physical fitness for women.
4. Mothers—Health and hygiene.   I. Shaw, Victoria.   II. Title.
RG801 .T75 2001
613.7'1'082—dc21   00-055210

ISBN 0-609-80554-1

10   9   8   7   6   5   4   3   2   1

First Edition

From Elizabeth

To my Lord and Savior Jesus Christ, who daily saves me

•

To my mother, Beverly Jean Chaney, who manages me from heaven's gate

•

To my children, Tatiana Lucillia, Lorenzo Lloyd, and Romeu William, who are constantly training me to be a strong mom by pushing me to my limits

•   •   •

From Victoria

To Camille and Julien, my true inspiration

Acknowledgments

FROM ELIZABETH

- To my dad, who reminds me how small the world is and how to roll around it

- To my sister, Carolyn Chaney, who has kept our mother's dream alive

- To Coty Sidnam, my first postpartum client, who continues to support my dreams

- To Dr. Henry Kissinger, who kept his dancer/trainer on her toes and rolling in the right direction

- To babyGap, for providing a place to gather before Strollercize classes and tons of support

- To Barbara Spector, who has kept me "grounded"

- To Victoria Shaw, who got the wheels turning on the book project

- To Judith Riven, who has been the most wonderful agent to Victoria and myself

- To Viktor Reign, who has "webbed" it all together for me

- To Arthur Julian and Gill King, the two talented photographers whose work adds so much to this book

- To the Strollercize moms who have participated since 1994. I look forward to Strollercizing when we are grandmas!

- To my Strollercize staff throughout the years, each believing in the mission and helping me to smile and laugh, even on the days I felt like "losing it"
- To the Strollercize moms and their babies who appear in this book—you all look *great,* I'm so proud of you
- To Antonio, the best father to our three angels!

FROM VICTORIA

I would like to thank my husband, Luc Faucheux, for his support, encouragement, and baby-sitting during the writing of this book, and my children Camille and Julien Faucheux, for sharing their mother with her computer for the past eighteen months. I would also like to acknowledge Yanne Menard for helping to keep my little ones occupied, and Jessica Pfeifer for always being there when I'm about to lose it. Finally, I would like to thank Elizabeth Trindade for teaching me how to Strollercize my way back into shape after the births of my two children, and for helping to make this mom's life just a little bit easier.

Contents

.... III ....

A Day in Your Life 151

Authors' Note

No matter what your age or current fitness level, anyone who participates in the Strollercize program, let alone any exercise program, must consult with her doctor, especially if she has any of these situations, which could affect working out:

- You have not participated in a regular fitness program in the past three to six months.
- You are overweight, or underweight, for your height and body type.
- You have been sedentary and have had little or no activity.
- You have a disease or chronic illness, including and not limited to, heart disease, diabetes, arthritis, high blood pressure, autoimmune disorders, and asthma.
- You are currently taking medication. Many drugs can affect your ability to work out.
- You have an injury, or chronic condition, that might be affected by exercising.
- You are pregnant, again!
- You have had dizzy spells or have felt light-headed.
- You are undergoing a lot of stress or are depressed and need additional help.

It is important to read every page of this book and to not skip exercises or chapters in performing the program. Go at your own pace and don't push yourself too hard. Fitness will come in time—be patient, be consistent, and use your common sense. If you have any questions or need additional fitness consulting, you may contact Strollercize at strollercize.com.

Introducing Strollercize

A SUPERMOTHER?

A new mother has a baby—and then disappears for three months. Where does she go, and what is she doing? She hides in her home, surrounded by baby gifts, afraid to venture out into her new world. She spends her days sitting in her rocking chair, feeding the baby, changing the baby, and scrubbing the spit-up stains off the couch. Her friends and family call with congratulations and ask how the delivery went. She answers in a broken voice, "We're doing fine. I just love being a mother." But she's lying. She feels all alone. She wants to be a supermom, but she feels like a failure. A big, shiny new stroller is parked near the door. She wonders if she will ever get it out of the house. Her husband comes home from work and asks about her day: "Did you have fun with the baby? Did you get out and see some friends?" She hands him the baby and runs out of the room crying. "I can't get out—I'm trapped!" That super-mom was me.★

WHAT IS STROLLERCIZE?

After the birth of my first child, Tatiana, I was "fitness frustrated." My body was fat, wide, and gushy. My life was out of control. As a former dancer and

★This book is written in the voice of Strollercize creator Elizabeth Trindade.

personal trainer, I was used to being in shape. But as a working mother, I didn't have much time for myself. Getting out of the house was a workout in and of itself, not to mention that the gyms in my area back then didn't have baby-sitting. I longed for the freedom I once had to work out when I wanted and to take care of my own needs. I wanted my life back! One night I took a lonely stroll with my big stroller. It was heavy and hard to push—and I was a trainer. Then the idea came to me: The baby's stroller is the perfect piece of exercise equipment. And the outdoors is the perfect gym. Strollercize was born.

Each day, a brigade of new mothers and infants file into parks and playgrounds all across New York City to whip their bodies into shape. Under the direction of certified Strollercize trainers, these newly inducted members of the "Motherhood" have discovered a workout routine designed especially for them. Strollercize offers new mothers a great way to get back in shape while being with their babies. You strap the baby into the stroller and take off for the park or the mall, or just stroll around the neighborhood. You don't have to spend a lot of money on a gym membership or hire a baby-sitter. The stroller and the baby become mom's weight-loss and resistance apparatus. Strollercize has helped me and thousands of other women reclaim their bodies and their lives. And it can help you too!

ABOUT THIS BOOK

Remember pregnancy? You read everything. Now that you are a mom, you barely have time to read a billboard. But please read this book. It will help. Keep this book in the diaper bag, or put it on top of that pile of magazines that has stacked up since the baby was born. Read a short section or two when you feed the baby, or when you're waiting in line at the supermarket. Just read it!

In this book, you'll learn a fun and effective exercise program specifically designed to meet the needs of new moms like you. With Strollercize, you're going to get your body back. You're going to increase your stamina, perk up your mood, and deal with the stresses of parenting. Following the "training for life" philosophy I developed as a personal trainer, you'll learn everything you need to know to make your new life a little more manageable. You'll learn how to maneuver your stroller in tricky situations, like doorways and crowded streets, and how to lift the baby without straining your back. You'll learn which muscles are most important to strengthen for motherhood and how to navigate the obstacle course that lies ahead of you and your stroller. Most importantly, you will increase your strength, endurance, and emotional well-being.

Strollercize helps you to feel good about yourself and your body as you train for the challenges of motherhood. When you are not doing the actual fitness routine, you can use the postures of Strollercize in your daily life. Approaching a curb, getting through a doorway, strolling to the playground, and standing in line at the grocery store to buy diapers all become opportunities to exercise. Whether you are a bit lazy or a fitness fiend, Strollercize can work for you. It is easy to adjust the intensity of the workout to meet your individual needs. And as the baby grows, so do the benefits of the Strollercize routine—the increased weight of your baby will increase the resistance of the stroller. This Strollercize routine will keep you strolling fit—with benefits that will last long after your baby outgrows the stroller. Welcome to Strollercize!

1
Welcome to Strollercize
. . . .

So you've made the commitment, and you're ready to start Strollercizing. The first five chapters of this book cover what you need to know to get started. In Chapter 1, I'll discuss the challenges of new motherhood and how Strollercize can help. Chapter 2 covers the basic ingredients of physical fitness. Chapters 3 and 4 offer tips for selecting the right stroller, dressing for success, finding your perfect stroller posture, and staying safe while strolling. Finally, Chapter 5 introduces the Strollercize Waist Away routine, which is guaranteed to firm up your midsection and strengthen your pelvic floor muscles. For best results, you should do this routine every day. Be sure you've mastered this routine before you move on to the complete Strollercize workout in Part II.

Congratulations! You're in the 'Hood . . . Motherhood

*Y*ou're exhausted, covered with spit-up, and desperate to fit into your old jeans. Welcome to motherhood. If you thought being a mom was going to be easy, think again. In fact, motherhood is one of the greatest physical and emotional challenges that you will ever face. The good news is that the rewards of being a mom make it all worthwhile.

THIS NEW LIFE

No matter how many books you read or classes you took while you were pregnant, nothing can truly prepare you for motherhood. From the moment you first hold your baby in your arms, your life will never be the same again. In the first few weeks with my firstborn, Tatiana, I felt as if my life had been turned inside out and upside down. There were new schedules to follow, new routines to adjust to, and so many new responsibilities. Plus, I was completely drained from around-the-clock feedings and the inevitable sleepless nights.

With everything you're going through, it's normal to feel a little bit overwhelmed in these early days of motherhood. You're tired, you're cranky, you're disoriented—but you can do it, Mom. Let Strollercize be your solution. Here's a rundown on how Strollercize can help you to cope with your new life.

Sleep Deprivation. Sure, I expected some sleepless nights after the baby was born, but not every night. Not only did Tatiana want to feed every ten minutes, but she also wanted to be held through the night. The truth is that unless you have twenty-four-hour child care and a wet nurse, you can't expect to get much sleep in those early weeks.

I know that after staying up half the night, the last thing you feel like doing is breaking a sweat. But do it anyway. Working out will actually give you more energy. How else do you think I manage to keep up with my three kids?

Mood Swings. Like most new moms, after my daughter was born, I was an emotional time bomb. My husband was walking on eggshells, certain that the next thing he did would be the wrong thing. What was the right thing? Who knew!

Sleep deprivation, hormonal fluctuations, a huge list of things to do—you are needed every second of the day, and you're expected to do ten things at once. You are doing a balancing act, and you can't balance. This can make you especially vulnerable to depression. In fact, an estimated 50 to 75 percent of new mothers experience some degree of postpartum depression. Don't be afraid to talk about these feelings. Seek out another mom, a close friend, or your husband. And get moving. A regular program of exercise can help fight depression.

Social Life. Been out of the house lately? Why is it that so many new moms hide at home? They dress their babies up in those cute little outfits, while they hang out in their sweatpants, afraid to be seen by even the mailman. Sound familiar? Then get out of the house! After "nesting" with the baby for days on end, even the most enthusiastic new mother is bound to go stir-crazy.

Believe me, I know what you're going through. All of your childless friends are going out at night and having fun. They want to meet for cocktails and talk about the places they've been and the movies they've seen. You haven't had time for a movie in months (not even on video), and you'd rather discuss more "important" topics like your baby's feeding and sleeping schedule. Don't worry, eventually you and your old friends will rediscover some common ground. In the meantime, try to make friends with other new moms.

Postpartum Depression

For an estimated 10 to 20 percent of new mothers, the baby blues turns into a full-blown case of postpartum depression. And some women get so down, they don't even realize they need help. Symptoms of postpartum depression include:

- *Incapacitating anxiety*
- *Insomnia, or excessive sleepiness*
- *Long periods of uncontrollable crying*
- *Mental confusion*
- *Loss of interest in grooming and personal hygiene*
- *Negative feelings toward your baby*

Postpartum depression is a serious condition and can interfere with your ability to care for your baby. If you think you may have more than a mild case of the blues, talk with your doctor or therapist.

Sex Life. Yep, having a baby means that your marital life is going to change too. Here's a sensitive situation. Some husbands get really romantic right after the baby. Do you blame them? Chances are, they haven't had sex for months. Now that the baby is out, they figure all systems are go! But as far as you're concerned, those "systems" are closed for renovation. Other men are terrified to touch their wives for months (or even years) after childbirth. Who knows what they're thinking? Maybe they're having trouble seeing Mom as a sex object, or maybe they're worried about damaging those still-fragile private parts.

After the delivery, doctors usually suggest that you abstain until the first checkup or six weeks. You'll thank your doctor for her or his sound advice. It's normal not to want to have sex after having a baby. After all, it's hard to feel romantic when you're sleep deprived and your body is not your own. Plus, you've got all those postpartum hormones working against you, especially if you're breast-feeding. While there are no magic spells to jump-start your sex life, Strollercize can help. Not only will the exercises increase your stamina, but pretty soon you'll feel more sexy with your buff new body.

THIS NEW BODY

If you've made it home from the hospital without passing by a full-length mirror, consider yourself lucky. Chances are that you won't exactly love what you see. A few weeks after having the baby, my husband and I wanted to go to a movie to celebrate our new family. After vainly searching my closet for an outfit, I finally collapsed in tears. How could I go out in public with this deformed body? My flesh was the consistency of Jell-O, and everything jiggled when I moved. My breasts were bigger than a porn star's, and my butt looked like the "before" picture in an ad for cellulite cream. I wanted to take the baby with me everywhere I went as an excuse for looking the way I did.

The fact is that most women leave the hospital looking like they did when they were six months pregnant. Then again, why would you expect anything different? Your body has taken a serious beating. After nine months of growing and stretching to accommodate the baby, it's going to take at least nine months for your body to recover its prebaby form. If you dare take a look in the mirror, be prepared for the following:

Your Abdomen. If you're like most new moms, the first thing that you'll notice is the sorry state of your midsection. The skin that was smooth and taut during your pregnancy is now droopy and wrinkled. And that glob of flesh underneath has the consistency of Play-Doh.

Strengthwise, your abdominal muscles are at ground zero. They're so weak that getting up out of bed may be more difficult than doing those prepregnancy abdominal crunches. And your weak, stretched-out abs may not be up to one of their most important tasks: supporting your lower back. As a result, many women experience lower back pain after the baby is born (see page 25). For some women, the abdominal muscles stretch so much that they end up separating down the center of the abdomen. This condition is known as diastasis recti, and most sufferers don't even know they have it. The bad news about diastasis is that it means you're getting even less support for your lower back. In Chapter 5, I'll say more about diastasis and show you a simple test for this condition.

No matter how severe the damage, with a little time and a lot of effort your belly will return to its former self (or close enough). The Strollercize abdominal routine in Chapter 5 will help.

Your Hips. After Tatiana was born, I was certain that I'd never again manage to get my hips through a narrow door frame. During your pregnancy, you too may have noticed that your hips started spreading like wildfire. You can thank the hormone relaxin, which works during pregnancy to loosen you up to make room for your growing baby. Relaxin stays in your bloodstream for up to six months postpartum. So you may have to forget about those tight skirts and narrow doorways for a while. To get rid of that flabby stuff on the outsides of your hips quicker, you'll need to Strollercize.

Your Pelvic Floor. Here's an important lesson: Do not sneeze, cough, or let anyone tell you a good joke until you have mastered the technique of "holding it." Yep, stress incontinence (i.e., leaking urine when you cough, laugh, or sneeze) is one of those postpartum surprises that nobody talks about. This happens because the muscles of the pelvic floor (PF) are weakened from the stress of pregnancy and childbirth. The PF muscles are very important—they support the contents of your pelvis, and they play an important role in sexual enjoyment. Weak PF muscles can cause problems during exercise, as you may leak when you run, jump, or even walk briskly. Wear protection, and "hold it" during high-impact movements. Chapter 5, which includes a great series of exercises to target these muscles, will come in handy for this tightening move.

Experts estimate that at least half of all postpartum women have some degree of laxity of the pelvic floor, with or without symptoms. And the problem may worsen over time and with each pregnancy. Whether you're leaking or not, you need to be strengthening your pelvic floor muscles as soon as possible.

Your Feet. Sorry, Cinderella—but there's no way you're fitting into that glass slipper anytime soon. If you were one of the many women whose feet swelled up three sizes during pregnancy, don't expect them to shrink back to normal right away. I gained a full shoe size with each of my pregnancies. But at least I had an excuse to buy some new shoes!

Even if your feet didn't grow during pregnancy, you may have to get used to using them again. It seems that after months of not being able to see their own feet, many moms simply forget they're still there. Besides, thanks to relaxin, your arches are flatter, your ankles are floppy, and your shins are weak. In the late stages of pregnancy, you may have waddled when you walked and did not use your feet in a proper stride. This can cause your toes, your ankles, and the arches of your feet to become stiff and weak.

Your Body Image. In a culture where svelte supermodels and movie stars are worshiped like goddesses, your postpartum figure can be hard to take. But remember, your body did a miraculous thing. You should feel proud. And speaking of superstar moms—you know why they always seem to emerge from childbirth with perfect bods? They have high-priced personal trainers, live-in chefs and nutritionists, and around-the-clock child care.

Famous or not, every mom has a job ahead of her. Some women may lose weight faster than others, but every mom has to work to regain her strength, stamina, and endurance. Be patient with yourself. With a little time and effort, you will surely be able to Strollercize your body back into shape.

MOTHERHOOD'S LABOR PAINS

As if pregnancy and childbirth did not do enough damage to your body, motherhood can also take a serious physical toll. I'm talking about the aches and pains from lifting the baby, carrying the baby, feeding the baby, bathing the baby, and last but certainly not least, pushing the baby in the stroller. New moms are especially susceptible to injury because their bodies haven't fully recovered from pregnancy and birth.

After each of my three childbirths, I felt pains in areas that I had no idea could even be injured. The prenatal classes prepared me for the birth, but none of the instructors said anything about how I would feel after the delivery. Actually, some of my worst "labor pains" surfaced long after the baby was born. Allow me to clue you in to some of the body parts that can be wounded on the battlegrounds of motherhood.

Shin Splints. If you've ever experienced that burning sensation up the front of your lower legs, you know firsthand how even a mild case of shin splints can ruin your day. This painful condition stems from poor posture, which is often worsened by pregnancy and motherhood. Another big "shin buster" is inactivity. If you slowed down (or stopped moving) during pregnancy, it may take some time for your shins to spring back into shape.

You can prevent shin splints by walking tall, wearing proper footwear, and always warming up these muscles before strolling (see Chapter 6).

Knee Pain. Chances are, your knees have had it. Due to the weak leg muscles and joint laxity brought on by pregnancy, your knees are probably not as stable as they once were. Plus, with the new baby, you're doing a lot of sitting, standing, bending, lowering, and lifting. Your baby's weight (and your own) puts a lot of stress on your knees. The exercises in Chapter 8 will help strengthen your quadriceps muscles to protect your fragile knees.

Lower Back Pain. If you've managed to make it through pregnancy and early motherhood without suffering from lower back pain, you are blessed and a rare case. Back pain is the number one complaint of new mothers. Just think about it—your growing baby put pressure on your spine for nine months. And now your weakened abdominal muscles aren't up to the task of stabilizing your spine. Then there's the poor posture, the widened hips, and the swollen feet. If you think you're strong enough for daily activities like bending over the changing table, carrying the baby, or loading the stroller into the trunk of the car—think again. Get started training your muscles to meet these daily challenges.

Upper Back Pain. While you're holding, cuddling, and kissing this miracle gift, your shoulders round and fall forward. You're feeling the joy of motherhood. But your upper back is not feeling so joyous. Here's a test: When you walk past the mirror, do you see a proud, erect mom or the Hunchback of Notre Dame's wife? If your back is rounded over and your head is on the same level as your shoulders, then you're asking for trouble. In the chapters that follow, I'll show you how to straighten up and put your head back on your shoulders.

Shoulder Strain. Motherhood is full of twists and turns. Getting your stroller through doorways, reaching for the toy that rolled under the couch, and securing your baby in his car seat can all involve physical contortions that even the most advanced yoga master wouldn't attempt. It's no wonder that many new parents wind up straining their shoulders. Add to this the fact that most new moms don't have the arm strength to lift and carry their babies. Once again they call on their shoulder muscles, and you have an injury waiting to happen. In Chapter 10, I'll show you how you can carry out your daily activities without straining your shoulders.

Wrist Pain. Wrist pain (like carpal tunnel syndrome and tendinitis) often surfaces in the last few months of pregnancy and can persist for months after the baby is born. New moms are especially sensitive to this annoying arthritislike pain. This condition is due to fluid retention, as well as the demands of the mother's daily life. Holding the baby, bottle feeding, and pushing the stroller can make the problem even worse. Proper body mechanics, wrist-strengthening exercises, and wrist braces can help.

Tennis Elbow. Even if you've never picked up a racquet, as a new mom you are especially vulnerable to tendinitis in the elbow, or tennis elbow. Surprisingly, the main culprit may be your stroller. Too many moms neglect to maintain proper elbow position when pushing the stroller. Other culprits include opening cans, yanking on big doors, and holding the baby. After a while, your elbow forgets which way it's supposed to hinge. No matter the cause, the results can be very painful.

Stiff Neck. Yes, your baby is beautiful. And yes, you could spend the entire day looking down into those tiny button eyes. But too many new moms walk around as if their chins were glued to their chests. The result can be a very stiff neck. Other neck stiffeners include anxiety, tension, and scrunching your shoulders up to your ears as if to ask, why me? Your neck muscles need to be strong and flexible. Your neck should move freely atop your relaxed shoulders. My favorite saying to help my clients relax their necks and shoulders is "Show off that diamond necklace and be proud to be a mother." Immediately, Mom lifts up her head, a smile returns to her face, and she walks with a little more pride.

Headaches. You may feel like you're telling your husband, "I have a headache," every day, but he should know it's not just a lame excuse! After you have

Why Strollercize?

- *Lose fat*
- *Get toned*
- *Increase endurance*
- *Have more energy (i.e., feel less tired at the end of the day)*
- *Improve your posture*
- *Be prepared to meet daily challenges*
- *Boost your immune system*
- *Improve your cardiovascular fitness*
- *Sleep better*
- *Reduce the need for a baby-sitter*
- *Reduce the need for a gym*
- *Reduce back pain*
- *Get stronger (such as for carrying the baby)*
- *Improve your flexibility*
- *Avoid incontinence*
- *Relieve stress*
- *Take care of yourself*
- *Stay healthy for your family*
- *Set a good example for your children*
- *Feel better about yourself*

a baby, the hormones in your body are fluctuating, and this can cause increased headaches. My advice: Start strolling. Physical activity can help ward off headaches.

STROLLERCIZE TO THE RESCUE

I don't need to tell you that motherhood, while extremely rewarding, is no picnic. Fortunately, there's a simple solution to all (or at least most) of your problems: Strollercize! Working out will give you more energy so you can get by on less sleep. You'll burn fat and calories to shed those excess pounds. And you'll be strengthening and toning those body parts that were stressed or neglected during pregnancy. Strollercize will help you cope with the physical and emotional stresses of motherhood. Not only will you burn some calories and blow off some steam, but you'll know that you're doing something positive for yourself and the baby. So what are you waiting for?

2

Mom's Fitness Formula

Before the birth of my first child, I thought I was in pretty good shape. Although I gained thirty-three pounds, I still assumed that I'd be back in my old jeans a month after the baby was born. Boy, was I wrong! Six months postpartum, I looked like I was five months pregnant. The only jeans I could squeeze into were a full size bigger and had an elastic waistband.

The truth is that no matter what kind of shape you were in before the baby, getting back to your prepregnancy form is never easy. For most of us, it takes nine to twelve months to lose the weight—and that's if you exercise regularly and watch what you eat. In fact, the average new mom holds on to that last ten pounds, never making it back into her old jeans at all. But it doesn't have to be this way. Between my three pregnancies, I gained and lost ninety-nine pounds! How did I do it? In this chapter, I'll give you the secret ingredients to my formula for fitness.

INGREDIENT 1: KNOW THE FACTS

Knowledge is power. In order to get fit, you have to understand some basic facts about fitness. "Physical fitness" has to do with how efficiently your body (especially your muscles, lungs, and heart) does its job. A high level of fitness means that you're able to carry out your daily activities—lifting the baby, running up and down stairs, doing laundry, cleaning house—and still have the energy to take a power stroll, without getting fatigued! A low level of fitness means you work up a sweat just getting up off the couch.

The only way to get fit is to challenge your body through a regular program of exercise. Exercise forces your heart, lungs, and muscles to work harder. Your lungs have to handle more oxygen. Your heart has to pump harder to get more blood to your muscles. With time the whole system becomes more efficient, and you become more fit.

There are five components to physical fitness:

Aerobic Capacity (Cardiovascular Fitness). Aerobic or cardiovascular fitness is the ability to engage in sustained physical activity (like climbing a few flights of stairs or chasing your toddler around the playground). It reflects how well your heart and lungs work together to supply oxygen to your body when you exercise. A regular program of aerobic exercise can improve your circulation, strengthen your heart muscle, and help you blow off some steam. And of course, aerobic activity burns calories.

Muscular Strength. Strong muscles make for a stronger person—and it takes a lot of strength to be a mom. Training your muscles will help you meet the physical demands of motherhood while toning up those flabby parts. Muscle conditioning helps to raise your metabolism: The more muscle mass you have, the more calories you burn (even while you're sleeping). Increasing your muscle mass is even more important as you get older. Starting in her late twenties, the average woman loses about half a pound of muscle mass each year. Muscle conditioning can slow this process and keep you strong as your children grow.

Flexibility. Flexibility has to do with how limber and supple you are. And moms need to be flexible—in their bodies, in their minds, and in their lives. Stretching improves joint range of motion, reduces muscular tension, and decreases injuries. Plus, tight muscles can contribute to the aches and pains of motherhood (see Chapter 1).

Balance and Coordination. This is my favorite component of fitness. When you train a group of muscles to perform an activity, you become more efficient.

So for example, if you practice lifting your baby (and I know you're getting a lot of practice with this one), over time this basic life move should start to get easier. Many of the exercises in Strollercize are based on moves from your daily life called "functional" exercises. These exercises teach balance and coordination and will improve your ability to carry out your daily activities like closing the car door with your leg while holding your baby. These exercises will help you to perform like a power parent.

Weight Control. I don't want you to mistake thinness for fitness. But if you are heavier than what is healthy for your bones, heart, and muscles, then you may need to watch your weight. Excess weight can slow you down, stress your joints, and make you feel sluggish and tired. If you top off that great workout with a trip to the local fast-food joint, you're not going to get fit—you are going to get fat! In Chapter 11 I'll give you some tips for getting those calories under control.

The Strollercize program targets each of these components. You'll get a great aerobic workout while taking the baby for a ride in the stroller (see Chapter 7). Using the stroller for balance and resistance, you'll learn simple moves to strengthen your muscles (see Chapter 8). I'll also show you some stretches to increase your flexibility and to help you get a handle on your new life (see Chapter 9). Finally, many of the exercises are based on activities from the daily life of a new mom. Practicing these moves during your workout will help you to manage the physical demands of motherhood.

INGREDIENT 2: SET APPROPRIATE GOALS

If you're like most new moms, your number one fitness goal has something to do with fitting into your old dress size or finding that magic number on your bathroom scale. That's natural. Few moms like the way their bodies look after childbirth. But remember, fitness is more than what you see in the mirror. Maybe you'd like to have more energy, or to be able to carry the baby without feeling it in your back. And of course, one of the best reasons to exercise is to improve and maintain your health. Exercise has been associated with health benefits like lowering blood pressure, preventing osteoporosis and heart disease, and reducing the risk of certain kinds of cancer. So when you are defining your goals, try to look beyond weight loss and physical appearance. You'll be more likely to stick with your exercise program if you focus on how exercise makes you feel rather than how it makes you look.

In setting your goals, try to be realistic. You're not going to lose twenty pounds in a month, or be running five miles a day just weeks after the baby is born. Having these unrealistic goals will just set you up for failure if you're lucky—and a serious injury if you're not. Here are some examples of more attainable goals set by New York City Strollercize moms:

Lose five pounds in six weeks.

Fit into my prepregnancy clothes in six months.

Start eating a more nutritious diet and watch portions.

Stroll a mile a day.

Fit into my jeans in nine months.

Increase my energy so that I can last through my day.

Be able to touch my toes without feeling tight.

Be able to climb three flights of stairs without getting winded.

Feel comfortable wearing a sexy, short skirt to dinner.

Stop being afraid of food.

Be able to stay up with the baby at night and still have enough energy
    for the day.

Got the idea? Then write down your own list of goals. Be specific. Post it on the refrigerator or another place where you'll be sure to see it. And refer to your goals frequently to help you stay on track.

INGREDIENT 3: FIND FITNESS

If you sit on the sofa waiting for those pounds to melt away, you may be sitting for the rest of your life. And even if you're one of those lucky moms who lose all of the weight without even trying (yeah, right), you'll still have to contend with that squishy belly and those jiggling thighs. If you want your body back, you'll have to find fitness in your life. Yes, your Strollercize workout will help you to burn excess calories, tone your trouble spots, and give you the energy to get through your day. But Strollercize is only the beginning. The key to fitness is to find ways to keep moving.

- **Walk instead of drive.** Just because you own a car doesn't mean you have to use it. If you have to get somewhere that's only a few minutes' drive from home, why not stroll there instead? Here in the Big Apple, most people don't even own cars. And the average New York City mom walks at least thirty minutes a day. That may explain why so many people gain weight when they move to the suburbs.

- **Park a few blocks away.** Are you one of those people who drive from one end of the parking lot to the other, trying to find a closer spot? Shame on you! Walk the extra distance to work, to the mall, or to your friend's house. You'll save the time and aggravation of searching for a parking spot. You'll also get a great workout.

- **Pick up your pace.** Wherever you are and whatever you're doing, try to do it with gusto. Don't creep through the mall like a turtle—speed up, use those legs, and take the opportunity to burn more fat.

- **Take the infant swing back to the store.** Yes, babies love motion. But carrying your baby or taking her for a stroll is a far better workout for you than sitting on the couch and watching her swing back and forth. And for an even better workout—stroll to the playground and push your baby in the swing. Great arm work!

- **Dance with the baby.** Turn up your favorite music, and let your house be your private disco. Hold the baby as you rock and roll. If it is nap time, try waltzing your little one to sleep. You can also use these dance moves as part of the warm-up for your Strollercize workout (see Chapter 6).

- **Clean the house.** You're going to hate this. But cleaning house burns calories. I clean my house and love every minute because I know I'm getting a great workout. Plus, for some reason babies just love watching Mom make the beds and scrub the floors. Hopefully someday they will join in and help!

• **Hand-wash the laundry.** Doing the laundry by hand (all those "onesies" pile up) is a great workout for your arms, trust me—I had no washing machine at one point. It's also a great way to let out some aggression.

INGREDIENT 4: MIND YOUR MINUTES

An occasional stroll won't do it. If you want to be fit, you'll have to put in the time. The American College of Sports Medicine recommends at least twenty minutes of aerobic exercise three times a week, plus fifteen minutes of muscle conditioning two or three times a week. Of course, as a working mother, I know how difficult it can be to find twenty seconds, let alone twenty minutes. And five times a week—well, Mom, those days are over! That's why I developed a fitness routine that is realistic for a mother's lifestyle. All you need is forty-five minutes (that includes warm-up, aerobics, muscle conditioning, and stretching) twice a week, and you'll see some serious results.

Of course, if you can make more time for exercise, then go ahead and splurge! Just don't overdo. Remember, the point of working out is to improve the quality of your life. Exercise should make you feel healthy, energetic, and relaxed. If you feel tired or stressed about your workouts, it's time to reevaluate your goals.

INGREDIENT 5: DON'T RUSH

Some moms are ready to start moving just moments after birth. The baby hasn't even cracked his first smile, and they're out training for their next marathon. Obviously, these moms are a bit overanxious! Even if you were active during pregnancy, you should still take a break after the baby is born. *The American College of Obstetricians and Gynecologists recommends that women wait at least six weeks postpartum before engaging in any vigorous exercise (longer if you had a difficult delivery or a C-section).* I couldn't agree more. Motherhood is a big adjustment, both mentally and physically. You need time to get used to your new life, and your body needs time to heal. Don't make yourself crazy by rushing things.

But there is one group of exercises that should absolutely be practiced as soon after delivery as possible: the pelvic floor exercises in Chapter 5. Otherwise enjoy this special time with your new baby.

After six weeks, with your doctor's okay, you'll be ready to start Strollercizing. During the first few weeks of your program, be sure to start slowly and increase gradually. Begin with short walks at a comfortable pace, plus a few gentle exercises to strengthen your pelvic floor and abdominal muscles (see Chapter 5). Be careful with high-impact activities like kick-boxing and running, because your joints are unstable. As you start to feel stronger, you should be able to handle the full Strollercize routine.

. . . .

Warning Signs

Sometimes in fitness even the best program can be too much. And as a new mom, you have to be especially careful because your body is still recovering from pregnancy and birth. Be aware of the following warning signs:

Heavy Bleeding. Some women experience a slight increase in vaginal bleeding after exercise. If you do, you should check with your doctor to make sure you're completely healed. You should contact your doctor immediately if you experience copious (i.e., soaking a pad every half hour), bright red bleeding that persists for several hours, or if you pass large clots of blood.

Pain. Exercise, especially in those first few weeks, should feel good. If it hurts, stop. Pain means that there might be something wrong and you should talk to your doctor.

Dizziness. Dizziness could mean many things. So again stop exercising, sit down, and wait for the feeling to pass. If possible, try to get someone's attention, as dizziness can lead to fainting. When your head clears, try to evaluate the situation. Are you overheated? Have you eaten enough? Could you be anemic? If these dizzy spells persist, see your doctor.

Chest Pain or Difficulty Breathing. It could be indigestion, but why take a chance? Stop exercising and get to a doctor.

Breast Infection or Abscess. If you experience pain or a lump in your breast, fever, or flulike symptoms, you may be suffering from a breast infection or abscess. Your doctor will suggest the best time to start exercising again. Stop exercising until the infection or abscess has cleared up completely. Vigorous movement can spread the infection.

. . . .

INGREDIENT 6: DON'T BE AFRAID TO BREAST-FEED

Breast-feeding can play an important role in a fit and healthy lifestyle. The average lactating mom produces almost a quart of milk each day—and uses an extra five hundred calories in the process. You may not see the results right away, but in the long run breast-feeding burns more calories, and moms are more likely to take off the weight quickly when they stop breast-feeding. Breast-feeding can also ease postpartum depression and reduce your risk of developing breast and ovarian cancer later in life. And the hormones released while you nurse help you feel more relaxed, while shrinking your uterus back to its former size.

Some people believe that exercise and breast-feeding don't mix. I'm not one of them. We hold regular "breast-feeding conventions" after Strollercize classes, and I have never heard a single complaint. Still, rumors persist. Here are some typical concerns.

Milk Supply. The number one concern of most nursing mothers is that exercise will affect their milk supply. But recent research suggests that regular exercise does not affect a nursing mom's milk supply. For the many years women have been Strollercizing, there has not been one complaint from the babies who have bellied up to Mom's breast.

Sour Milk. You may have heard that exercise can make your breast milk taste sour. Indeed, a few studies have found increased levels of lactic acid in breast milk following periods of intense exercise. Lactic acid is not dangerous to the baby, but it can temporarily make your milk taste sour. Other studies, however, have failed to find similar effects.

Milk Quality. Some studies say vigorous exercise temporarily (i.e., for about one or two hours after a workout) decreases the immunity benefits of breast milk. As a result, some experts recommend that you wait an hour after exercise before breast-feeding. After Strollercize, those babies do not want to wait an hour! Before you get too concerned, do keep in mind that the average three-month-old baby nurses about six to eight times a day. Chances are your baby will get an adequate boost to her immunity from those other five to seven feedings.

I see absolutely no reason why the average nursing mom should not exercise. Of course, this is not to say that you shouldn't be careful. For instance, if you notice that your baby rejects the breast after you exercise, try feeding her before you work out. (This is a good idea regardless, because it's uncomfortable to exercise with full breasts.) And while exercise shouldn't affect your milk supply, your doctor will monitor your baby's growth and development, making sure your little one grows into a big guy! Finally, breast-feeding moms need extra calories and fluids to make up for what they expend during exercise. You should be especially careful to drink enough fluids, and always be on the lookout for the following signs of dehydration:

- Dry mouth
- Fatigue
- Excessive thirst
- Dark, scanty urine
- Dizziness
- Muscle cramps

INGREDIENT 7: COMMIT TO BE FIT

Sure you'd love to go for a midmorning jog, cook a low-fat dinner, and then take an evening stroll with your family. Too bad you haven't got the time. You have play group in the morning, a doctor's appointment in the afternoon, and absolutely no food in the house. Face it: You'll probably end up ordering a pizza and camping out in front of the TV.

Being a mom is hard work. There will always be chores to do, places to go, and people to see. But if you want to get fit, you'll have to make the commitment. Physical fitness is a state of mind: Fit people respect themselves and their bodies. They make the time to exercise because their health and well-being are top priorities.

Some women love to exercise. Others do it because they know they should. But most new moms give up on exercise because they lack the will to continue. In fact, only 3 percent of all new moms maintain a regular workout schedule after having a baby. That leaves 97 percent of you with weight to lose, wearing big baggy pants and an oversize T-shirt, slumped over a stroller and pushing it with low self-esteem and no energy. This mom I define as the "mall mom," and she is the mom I care about the most. Are you a mall mom? If you are, don't panic. Strollercize is going to help you change your lifestyle because exercise is easy and fun to do. Soon you will be shopping with a strut and passing other moms with new energy and a swing at your local mall! Go, girl!

.... 3 ....

Equipped to Strollercize

You've got the car seat, changing table, baby carrier, and diaper bag. Then there are the clothes for days, clothes for nights, the high chair, the bouncy seat, and of course, the stroller. If you're like most new moms, you've got a house full of baby gear, and you're starting to wonder, Do I really need all of this stuff? Indeed, some of these things can help make your life easier. But too much stuff can weigh you down. In this chapter, I'll show you the essential equipment for the Strollercizing mom.

THE STROLLER

In the gym, there are treadmills, stair climbing machines, and rowing machines. In your life, there is the stroller. The stroller is the perfect piece of exercise equipment. It provides plenty of resistance, doubles as a balance bar, and even seats a tiny audience. But you need to choose your stroller carefully. The right stroller can be a mom's best friend; the wrong stroller—her worst enemy.

When I was pregnant with Tatiana, I received the gift of a gorgeous antique baby carriage. It was big, and no, I couldn't fold it up if I needed to jump in a taxi, but it looked so beautiful parked in our foyer. The carriage seemed like the perfect gift—that is, until the baby was born. You see, we lived in a six-story walk-up apartment. To leave the house, I had to carry that twenty-pound carriage (not to mention the baby) up and down six flights of stairs. Needless to say, I didn't get out much.

Which Stroller Is Right for You?

Strollers have different names: buggies, carriages, prams, push chairs, umbrellas, convenience, portable, double, side-by-side, tandem, and travel systems. Some sit, and some stand. Some are car seats, and some turn into car seats. Some have three wheels. No wonder shopping for a stroller can be as overwhelming as choosing a name for the baby. Each type of stroller has its own unique advantages and disadvantages, and none is even close to perfect. Maybe that's why the average family purchases four strollers before they settle on the one that suits their needs.

I have owned more than twenty-two strollers, and I've seen hundreds more in my classes. Allow me to share some of my wisdom. Let's start with the basic models.

Carriages or Prams. A carriage (pram) is that big, beautiful, and very expensive stroller with which you might imagine yourself casually strolling in the garden on a sunny spring day. It may be a family heirloom, or it may be shiny and new. Aside from their grace and beauty, carriages are sturdy, comfortable for the baby, and tend to have huge baskets for storing everything you need to take with you on your outings and then some. I love them in the winter because they offer great protection from the wind, snow, and rain. Carriages are best for newborns, who want to be fully reclined while strolling. Some models come with special seats for older babies, who prefer to sit up.

The main disadvantage of baby carriages is that they are huge, heavy, and difficult to maneuver (especially in tight spaces). More important, perhaps, is that they cannot be folded. This can be a serious problem if you want to put the stroller in the trunk of your car or bring it with you to a cozy restaurant. If you choose a pram, you'd better be doing some serious weight lifting. The average weight of this type of stroller is about twenty-eight pounds, not including the added weight of the baby, his toys, the diaper bag, and your shopping bags!

I am not a big fan of oversize baby carriages because they really slow you down. But if your heart is set on a fancy carriage, don't let me stop you. Just know what you're getting yourself into.

Convertible Strollers. Convertibles are the workhorses of strollers, as they are designed to be used for both infants, who must recline, and older babies and toddlers, who usually prefer to sit upright. Many convertible models have adjustable handlebars so that you can choose between having the baby face toward you while you stroll (great for younger babies) or letting her look out at the road ahead.

All in all, convertible strollers are a good option for cost-conscious parents (although some models can be as expensive as carriages) because you don't have to buy a separate infant stroller and umbrella stroller (see below). On the downside, convertible strollers tend to be less comfortable for the baby than carriages and much bulkier than umbrella strollers. And even if you buy a convertible stroller initially, you may still decide to buy an umbrella stroller when the baby is older, for the sake of convenience.

Umbrella Strollers (Convenience Strollers). These strollers get their name because they are intended to be folded up and carried like umbrellas when not in use. Good luck! The average umbrella stroller weighs ten to seventeen pounds. And though it would be nice to have a stroller that could be folded and unfolded as simply as an umbrella, it rarely works out this way. Most umbrella strollers require both hands to fold, and many require that you take your body through strenuous moves like a lunge and bending forward to fold them.

The main disadvantage of umbrella strollers is that most of them do not fully recline to 180 degrees, and are therefore appropriate only for older babies. If you decide to go with an umbrella stroller, you may still need to purchase a carriage or convertible stroller—which can get expensive.

Despite their limitations, I do love these strollers. They are much smaller, lighter, and easier to maneuver than carriages and convertible strollers. And they are essential if you ever want to take your baby into a crowded store, visit a friend who lives up a few stairs, or take some form of public transportation. My favorites are the new high-quality models that fully recline (making them suitable for babies of all ages). These are great for the active mom, and they really give you the best of both worlds.

Travel Systems (Car Seat Strollers). The newest addition to the stroller market is the combination car seat/stroller. If you hate having to transfer your sleeping baby from the car seat to the stroller (and vice versa) without waking him, you may be aching for one of these. The basic design is simple. The baby rides in a "portable" car seat that is attached to the stroller. Once the baby outgrows the car seat, the stroller converts into a front-facing, nonreclining stroller.

The main problem with the stroller/car seat combo is that it encourages parents to use the car seat as a baby carrier. But carrying a baby in a car seat is like lifting a fifteen-pound dumbbell (if the baby is a newborn)! Unless you've been training with some serious weights in the gym, you'll be nursing an injury and a baby!

Jogging Strollers (Three-Wheelers). God bless Yakima Washington who invented the Baby Jogger! Jogging strollers are great for the active and fit family. They glide across the ground and give the baby a supersmooth ride. But most models are not suitable for newborns because they do not fully recline. And they do not fold easily or compactly. Finally, since they tend to be huge and difficult to maneuver, they can't be used in place of an everyday stroller. (You'll still have to buy another stroller for everyday use.) The bottom line: If having a jogging stroller appeals to you, go for it! I stand behind any product that encourages mothers to exercise. But remember, you don't *need* a three-wheeler to do Strollercize.

Double Strollers. If you have twins or two young children, a double stroller is probably your only option. There are two basic types: tandem and side-by-side. With the tandem models, one child sits in front of the other (although some have adjustable seats so that the children can also face each other). Because they are narrower, tandem models are easier to maneuver and are more likely to fit into tight spaces (although they are considerably longer than single-occupancy strollers). Some parents also prefer to keep the children separated to minimize fighting en route.

Fans of side-by-side models like the fact that their children are sitting next to each other, where they can interact. These models also avoid disagreements about who gets the "front seat." Some New York City moms say that it's easier to get over curbs with a side-by-side stroller. But I have no idea how they manage to fit those things into all those tiny stores and restaurants. In some cases, side-by-sides do not fit through single doors! And side-by-side models can be hard on your shoulders. I know, because I pushed a side-by-side for two years.

One last thing. If you end up using a double stroller, you must be sure that your body is prepared. After all, that fully loaded stroller could easily weigh upward of sixty-five pounds or more, and you'd better be strong enough to push it. Here's where the Strollercize workout will really come in handy. In fact, if you don't work out, I guarantee that your body will give out long before your kids outgrow the stroller.

Shopping Tips

No matter what type of stroller(s) you decide to go with, there are a few basic things that you should look for.

Stability. You do not want that stroller to tip over. Put your diaper bag on the stroller, and then shake it, try to tip it, and see if it stays standing. A stable stroller should have a long, wide wheel base, and the seat should sit low and deep in the stroller's frame. The stroller should resist tipping backward if you push down on the handlebar: try it out, or put your bag on the back of the stroller, and see if it tips back.

Good Braking System. The stroller's brakes should have a double-locking mechanism. Check them out. Are they easy to use? Does the stroller still roll a little when the brakes are engaged? If it does, it's no good. I'm sure you'd like to avoid a runaway stroller!

Smooth Ride. The stroller should have good suspension, which you can feel if you take it for a test drive (see page 45). Here's a test: Put a toy in the stroller, and go for a stroll. If the toy falls over easily, then there's too much vibration. The seat should be well padded and shaped to support the baby's delicate spine. Some strollers will give a little bit when you shake them. Not to worry—this is how they absorb the shock of the ride for the baby.

Reliable Restraining Belts. Just imagine how you'd feel if your baby tumbled out of her stroller. Your stroller should have a safe and reliable system for restraining her. (And always use it!) Lap belts and bars are okay. (Never rely on the bar alone—the baby can slip out underneath.) But I prefer models that also have a shoulder harness. The shoulder harness is especially important with the lighter umbrella strollers, which have a tendency to tip over backward.

Make sure that the restraining belts are securely attached to the stroller and that the space around the leg holes is not so large that the baby can slip out. The buckle should be easy for you to close but hard for the baby to undo. Some older babies do manage to escape from their strollers, which can be dangerous!

Durable, High-Quality Wheels. Right up there with safety is your baby's comfort while riding in the stroller. To avoid a bumpy or jarring ride, the stroller's wheels should be well cushioned and large enough to go over cracks, bumps, and curbs smoothly. I have seen and heard about a few tires going flat. The stroller should glide along (not vibrate).

Locking Mechanism. A good locking mechanism will prevent the stroller (convertible and umbrella models) from accidentally collapsing. Make sure that the stroller has a secondary safety latch to prevent it from accidentally collapsing on the baby. The safest models require two separate steps to close.

JPMA Certification. For added assurance that a stroller is safe, to see whether it is certified by the Juvenile Products Manufacturers Association (JPMA). Surprisingly, some of the most popular and costly models do not have JPMA certification.

Lightness. The average stroller weighs about 22 pounds. (The range is between 7 and 30 pounds.) Add to that an overstuffed diaper bag (approximately 2 to 3 pounds), a few shopping bags (4 pounds), and your baby (the average six-month-old weighs about 14 pounds), and you might as well be pushing a cart of bricks! That's why when it comes to selecting a stroller, lighter is always better. Sure that 26-pound model may seem as safe as a tank. But tanks have engines, and strollers just have moms.

Ease of Folding. Unless you walk everywhere and plan never to use your car, ride the bus, or take the baby to a restaurant, you will need to be able to fold up your stroller. Accordingly, "easy to fold" should be high on your list of stroller criteria. The best choice is a stroller that can be folded with one hand, so that you can hold the baby while folding it. Also remember to choose a model with a secondary safety latch (see page 44).

Handlebars. Another important consideration when purchasing a stroller is the height of the handlebar(s). If the handlebar is too high or too low, you risk serious stress to your upper back, shoulders, and wrists. To test if a particular model is the right height for you, stand next to it (preferably facing a mirror), and rest your hands on the handlebar. Check out your form. Your arms should be bent at a 130-degree angle at the elbow, your shoulders relaxed, open, and down, and your back straight with your chest up. If your elbows are bent at a 90-degree angle, then the handlebar is too high for you. If, on the other hand, your arms are completely straight and your upper body is hunched down over the stroller, then the handlebar is too low. Don't forget to repeat this test with everyone who will be pushing the stroller (Mom, Dad, a caregiver). What may be perfect for Mom may be too short for Dad or vice versa. A few of the strollers on the market have adjustable-height handlebars. You can also purchase handle extensions for some strollers.

While we're on the topic of handlebars, I should tell you that I prefer strollers with one single bar to those with two separate handles. Maybe it comes from my years as a dancer holding on to that ballet bar. But I think that these handlebars are more comfortable and easier to maneuver and put less strain on the wrist joints.

The Test Drive

So you think you've found a stroller with all the necessary features? Before you leave the store, I recommend that you give that stroller a test drive. After all, you wouldn't buy a car without testing it out. Well, for the fit mom, your stroller may be your most important set of training wheels. Keep in mind that pushing an empty stroller in the store is very different from pushing the stroller with your baby down a street. To get an idea of how it will handle in the real world, test out the stroller with baby on board, or load it up with at least ten pounds of baby gear. And while you're at it, check out how the stroller handles as you move down the narrow aisles and around the tight corners of the store. Does the cargo bounce around in the stroller? Do the wheels tend to veer off in one direction? (Try pushing with just one hand.) Are the wheels too small to roll up and over curbs and rough terrain? With a good stroller, the answer should be no to all of the above.

Confused? I don't blame you. As I said before, there are no perfect strollers (although I'm working on developing one). The trick is to weigh the pros and cons to find the stroller(s) that will best meet your individual needs. If your house has a dozen porch steps, don't buy a heavy carriage that can't be folded and carried upstairs. If you spend a lot of time in the car, look for a stroller that will actually fit in your trunk. Whatever your needs, you should always choose function over form. A huge, antique carriage may make a great family heirloom, but if you can't load it into your car to go to the mall, what's the point? In my opinion, the best stroller is one that weighs less than ten pounds, can be folded with only one hand, has medium to large shock-absorbing wheels, and reclines for a sleeping baby. But the choice is yours.

YOUR STROLLERCIZE WARDROBE

The truth is, I don't care if you exercise in your birthday suit (that could also be motivational!) as long as you exercise. But the right wardrobe can help motivate you to reach your fitness goals. Dress like a "fit mom," and you might start to feel like one. Here are the essential components of your Strollercize wardrobe:

Shoes and Socks. You'll need a pair of comfortable, well-cushioned, and supportive shoes. "Cross trainers" (fitness shoes) are great. They allow you to move forward and sideways, and they give you good support in the arches. And cross trainers give you the flexibility to switch between different activities (from walking to body strengthening to dancing in your living room) without having to switch shoes.

Now, about that old pair of sneakers in the back of your closet—I suggest that you toss them! Remember, your feet may have grown during pregnancy. And the average life expectancy of fitness shoes is only three to six months. Wearing those old, worn-out shoes can lead to nasty injuries like shin splints. Do yourself a favor, and invest in some new shoes.

Finally, shoes aren't the only necessary equipment for those tender toes. A thick, cushy pair of socks will make a big difference in your stride, while preventing blisters. Since your feet sweat a lot in athletic shoes, go for breathable fabrics, designed to whisk away moisture.

Supportive "Sports" Bra. Next to your stroller, the second most important piece of equipment that you're going to need for your Strollercize workout is a supportive bra. Whether you're big busted or flat chested, a good bra is essential not only for your comfort but to avoid damaging your breasts. Those bouncing bosoms on the opening credits of *Baywatch* may get your husband's attention, but they're a bad idea unless you want your breasts to end up sagging down to your belly button.

If you're nursing, exercising without a serious sports bra won't even be an option. Your breasts will be so sore and full of milk that you may need a heavy-duty bra just to walk across the living room. Unfortunately, it's hard to find nursing bras that are supportive enough for even moderate exercise. And even specially designed sports bras are not supportive enough for many nursing moms. Your best bet is to double up: Two sports bras, or a sports bra worn over a nursing bra, will probably do the trick. The advantage of the latter is that if you're really talented, you can discreetly take off the sports bra when it's time to nurse.

Leggings or Loose Pants, and a Comfortable Top. Tight compresses the flab, but loose feels more free. Short keeps you cool, but you have to be brave. Black is the color of choice because it makes you look slim and conceals leaks. (If you have this problem, you know what I'm talking about.) But do try to add a brightly colored shirt or jacket so that you will be visible to traffic. Avoid anything that's 100 percent cotton or wool. Instead, opt for a fabric that is designed to absorb sweat. Breast-feeding moms will need easy access to the breasts. Yes, those long baggy T-shirts cover your buns, but the longer the shirt, the harder it is to get breast lunch for the baby. (If you are worried about public bun exposure, tie a long-sleeve shirt around your waist to cover your hips.)

It may be worth the extra few minutes to pick an outfit that you feel good about wearing. A high-tech top or a flattering pair of shorts can really boost your morale and help you stay motivated. Keep the comfortable clothes handy for your workout. As a mobile mom, you'll want to be prepared to get active whenever the opportunity arises. I know quite a few New York City moms (not

Strollercize moms, of course) who cannot walk more than a few blocks because their trendy new shoes and tight little outfits aren't made for movement. While you don't have to give up style completely, it pays to be prepared. Put on a pair of shoes that you can actually walk in. Select an outfit that allows you to move around. And dress in layers, so you won't get too warm if you decide to pick up the pace.

Gloves. Gloves give you a better grip and better control, and of course they come in handy in colder weather. Gloves keep your hands clean for emergency diaper changes, and they protect your skin from the sun. I prefer white gloves, just like the traffic cop, so that when I hold up my hand to stop a passing car, the driver can actually see it. "Strollercize driving gloves" are perfect for gripping the handlebars for controlling the stroller.

A Watch with a Minute Hand. This important piece of equipment comes in handy for timing the duration of your workout and checking your heart rate (see Chapter 7). Not to mention that a new mother's day can fly by, so check the time and keep a schedule (see Chapter 11).

Leak Protection. In the first months after the babies, I nearly bought "adult diapers," therefore taking the title "Queen of Incontinence." As spokeswoman for a number of Strollercize moms, I will say that your first days of moving and bouncing will cause little leaks, letting you know how weak your pelvic floor muscles have become. Don't be embarrassed. Just be sure to add protection pads to your underwear until you have regained control (see Chapter 5).

THE DIAPER BAG

I get nervous with the whole subject of diaper bags. I have seen many a mom come to class with what looks like a full-size suitcase hanging on her stroller! I always wonder, is she heading to the airport after class? The fact is that when it comes to loading the diaper bag, too many moms seem to forget that they're only driving to the supermarket, not hiking to Alaska. After packing a roomful of toys, two economy packs of diapers, and a week's worth of formula, most moms can barely lift their diaper bags, let alone carry them.

When packing your diaper bag, think light. You'll be surprised at how little you really need to be prepared for almost anything. Here's my suggested gear for the average, one- to two-hour outing (in order of importance):

Two Diapers and Some Wipes. You'll want to bring more, but don't. Babies don't poop as often as you think.

One or Two Bottles (for Formula-fed Babies). Even if you feed the baby before you leave the house (which I strongly recommend), you can never predict when his little tummy will be ready for more.

A Backup Clean Outfit for the Baby. This is essential if your baby's prone to spitting up or if there is a diaper leak. It's also nice to have a sweater, in case the weather surprises you or the air conditioner is blasting.

A Baby Blanket. This is a must all year round. It's great not only for protecting the baby from the elements but for propping, folding, and making her feel secure and comfy. You may even use it later for a picnic or as a prop in your abdominal workout.

Stroller Plastic (Depending on the Weather). If the weather is iffy, you'd better bring a plastic to shield the baby from wind, rain, and blowing debris. The last thing I want you to think is that you can't work out in the rain.

A Few Small Plastic Bags (Optional). Plastic bags are great for disposing of dirty diapers and storing wet cloths.

A Pacifier (Optional). I'll stay out of the debate over whether pacifiers are good for your baby. But if you're using a pacifier, you'll probably want to have one with you at all times. Secure it to the baby's outfit—I can't tell you how many pacifiers I have lost.

One or Two Small Toys (Optional). Watching Mom exercise should be stimulating enough. But if you must bring toys, think small and simple.

First-Aid Kit (Optional). This should include some adhesive bandages, antiseptic wipes, an ice pack, and an Ace bandage.

GEAR FOR MOM

When packing your gear, you think "Baby, baby, baby." Yes, the baby is important, but so are you! Make sure to leave room in your bag for these essential items:

A Bottle of Water and a Snack. I can't tell you how many moms come to Strollercize class without bringing a bottle of water! It's important for you to stay hydrated and well nourished, especially if you're breast-feeding. A small bottle of water, plus a piece of fruit or some whole-grain pretzels, should do the trick.

Sunglasses. No matter the season, if there's sun, you should be prepared with sunglasses. Bright sun can be blinding, and squinting can lead to excess wrinkles. You need to be able to see clearly around you. Many runners wear protective eyewear to keep insects and other flying debris out of their eyes. You and your little one should do the same.

Sunscreen. Put it on. If you are outdoors, you must protect your skin from those harmful rays. If you're not wearing gloves, don't forget your hands, which are completely exposed as they rest on that handlebar.

Cell Phone (for Emergencies). When cell phones first came out I saw plenty of New York City moms gabbing with husbands, setting up the play dates, and even making dinner reservations in the middle of Central Park. Truthfully, I thought it was ridiculous. But over the years, I've seen how a cell phone can calm a mom's nerves in a minor crisis—and be a lifesaver in an emergency.

Now that you know what you need, you're ready to stroll. But with all those postpartum hormones clouding your memory, don't be surprised if you forget a few things. The following checklist should help.

CHECKLIST

- ❏ Your stroller
- ❏ Comfortable clothes, shoes and socks, and leak protection (if necessary)
- ❏ Gloves

- ❑ Water bottle and snack for Mom
- ❑ Formula bottle and/or snack for the baby
- ❑ Stroller plastic (depending on the weather)
- ❑ Sunglasses
- ❑ Sunscreen
- ❑ Cell phone (to make an emergency call)
- ❑ Baby blanket
- ❑ Diapers and wipes
- ❑ The baby!

4

Ready, Set, Strollercize!

Strollercize is a serious physical workout. You will sweat. You will get results. You will feel great! In the chapters that follow, I'll show you how to turn a stroll with your baby into a serious workout. This chapter will discuss Strollercize training as well as how to chart your course toward a fit life.

POSTURE CHECK

Pushing a stroller takes a lot of muscle. Pushing the right way will give you a great workout, but pushing the wrong way could result in a serious injury. So before you even think about going for a stroll, understand the basics of your perfect pushing posture.

Take a look at the two pictures on page 53. Which one do you want to look like? I bet you didn't choose the one on the left. After all, her body language is not exactly screaming "friendly, happy mother." Her head is down, her eyes are glazed over, and her body is hanging over the stroller as if she's glued to it. Now, look at the same mom in the picture on the right. Her chin is up, her shoulders are square. Her stomach looks flatter, her upper body is strong, her chest is lifted, and her hips look more toned. She looks more confident, alert, energized, and proud to be a mom.

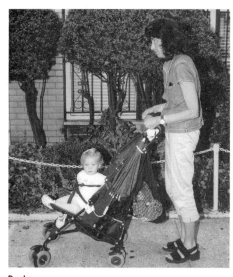
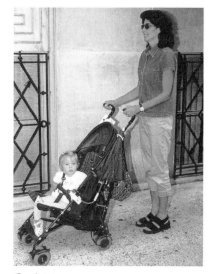

Bad posture   Good posture

With good posture, you won't just look better, you'll feel better too. Poor posture is a major contributor to the aches and pains of motherhood, including headaches, lower back pain, tennis elbow, and carpal tunnel syndrome (see Chapter 1). And since an active mom like you is likely to log in a lot of hours behind the stroller, it's important to find the right form.

To find the perfect pram-pushing posture, we Strollercizers say stand with an attitude like a movie star, lifted and pulled in, with an air of confidence. Are you laughing? Good—laughter tightens the abdominals and puts a smile on a new mom's face. Improving your posture may be the most important thing you do to make your new life more manageable and ensure your continued good health.

First, let's see how you measure up. To check out your posture, grab your stroller (or you can substitute the back of a chair), and stand in front of a full-length mirror. Then use the following list to see how you stand:

Your Feet. Your feet should always be closer together than the wheels of the stroller. Keep your feet close together and your knees under your hips. By bringing your legs closer to your midline, you will strengthen your lower back, minimize hip pain, and slim down your thighs. And remember, a wide stance only accentuates your already-widened hips.

Your Toes. Your toes should be pointing straight ahead, neither turned out nor turned in. Due to weak leg muscles and changes in their center of gravity during pregnancy, many women get in the habit of waddling, kind of like ducks, with their toes pointing outward. Unfortunately, the "duck walk" puts strain on your ankles and knees and can make your hips look much wider than they actually are. I can say this as a retired ballerina!

Your Knees. Your knees should face straight ahead and be directly under your hipbones. Because of weakened inner and outer thigh muscles, many new mothers walk with their knees internally rotated. If uncorrected, this knock-kneed stance can stress the knee joint.

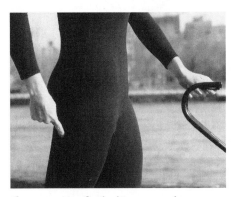
Correct position for the hips, rear, and tummy

Your Hips. Are you looking a little lopsided? Every mom has a favorite side for carrying the baby, breast-feeding, and hanging the diaper bag. With time, the muscles on the more frequently used side of your body grow stronger than the muscles on the less frequently used side. This muscular imbalance throws your spine out of alignment and can lead to lower back pain. When strolling, your hips should be square to the stroller and level with the handlebar. Imagine wearing a tight red leather skirt.

Your Rear End. You may not be loving the size of your butt, but don't try to hide it by tucking it under your torso. Tucking your pelvis overstretches the lower back muscles, causing your upper back and your abdominal muscles to weaken and your hamstrings to tighten. You're better off letting your bottom stick out a little bit, and keep your abdominals tight and lifted. Honestly, your bottom's not as big as you think.

Your Tummy. Tilt your head down, and look for your belly button. If you can see it over those extralarge breasts, then you have a problem (unless, of course, you're still pregnant). My point is that your stomach should be as flat as a board, not pooched out like a purse. I know, there's some extra you hanging around your midsection. But it will be a lot less noticeable if you keep your abdominal muscles pulled in tight (see Chapter 5). In fact, the main reason you've got that bulging belly is that your abdominal muscles are still weak. If you don't learn to pull in your tummy now, that potbelly could become permanent. You also risk developing chronic lower back pain.

Your Chest. Are your nipples dancing on your belly button? Not a great look! During pregnancy and nursing, the weight of your enlarged breasts tends to pull your body forward, especially if your upper back and chest muscles are weak. The result is slouching shoulders and sagging breasts. I know you're exhausted and your breasts weigh a ton. But for the sake of your posture (not to mention your morale), you should keep your chest lifted.

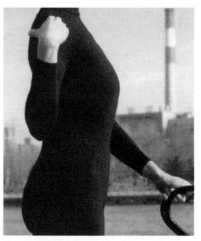

Correct position for the shoulders and chest

Your Shoulders. Are you wearing your shoulders as earrings? Well, scrunching up your shoulders will lead to a stiff neck and tight shoulders. Without constant attention to your form, nursing and cradling the baby, as well as pushing a heavy stroller, can exaggerate this poor, upper body posture. So invest in a diamond necklace, and keep your chest up and your shoulders relaxed and down!

Your Elbows. It takes a lot of effort to keep the muscles in the middle of your back strong and open. Most moms let their arms flop down by their sides. But this weakens the muscles of the middle back and shoulders. It also limits diaphragmatic (i.e., deep) breathing. So try to keep your elbows out. The extra energy in your upper torso will keep your arms toned and protect your elbows.

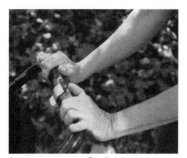

Incorrect position for the wrists

Your Wrists. Are you strangling your stroller? Gripping onto the handlebar for dear life can stress the wrist joints, let alone the elbow and neck. Another major stressor: bending your wrists when you stroll. Improper wrist position can lead to carpal tunnel syndrome and tendinitis of the wrists and elbows. So keep your hands relaxed and your wrists

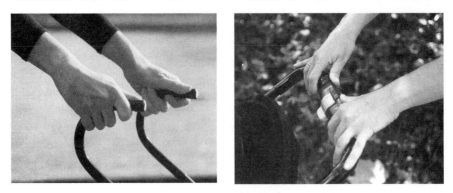

Correct positions for the wrists

straight, as in the photos (which show both a single handlebar stroller and a two-handled model).

Your Neck and Chin. While it's nice to look down at the baby from time to time, too many moms seem to be stuck in the chin-to-chest mode. The result: a double chin, a strained neck, a weakened upper back, and slumped shoulders. Don't hang your head. Keep your chin lifted and your neck wrinkle free.

Maintaining good posture takes constant thought and effort, and improving it takes time. When you Strollercize, you must keep fine-tuning your posture. The right way may feel like the wrong way until you get used to it. But good posture is worth getting used to. Of course, good posture also depends on strong and flexible muscles. That's why I've designed the Strollercize routine to train your muscles and correct common muscular imbalances.

I know I've given you a lot to remember. So, if your memory is not what it used to be, photocopy the Strollercize Posture Checklist (see page 57) and toss it in your diaper bag or tape it onto the stroller. Glance at the list from time to time, then check your form. Remember, keep your chest lifted and your shoulders down and relaxed. Your tummy should be pulled in tight. Keep your chin up and your toes facing forward. And keep smiling! Pretty soon you'll be pushing with strength, energy, and pride.

Strollercize Posture Checklist

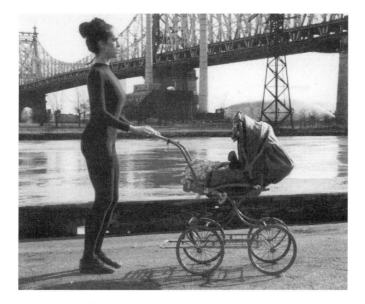

- ☑ Feet closer together than the wheels of the stroller
- ☑ Toes pointed straight ahead
- ☑ Knees pointed straight ahead
- ☑ Tummy pulled into spine
- ☑ Hips level
- ☑ Chest up
- ☑ Shoulders down and relaxed
- ☑ Chin lifted and neutral
- ☑ Elbows slightly out
- ☑ Wrists straight

CHARTING YOUR COURSE

You can do your Strollercize workout practically whenever and wherever you want: in the park, on the sidewalk, or even in the mall. You can even fit this routine into your regular activities, like going to the store or strolling through the neighborhood. When planning your workout, look for a location that will be stimulating for both you and the baby. Pleasant scenery and friendly faces can ease the boredom factor for both of you. For safety's sake, avoid strolling where there is heavy traffic, rough terrain (unless you have a heavy-duty, three-wheeled stroller), or other potential hazards. And be sure to make convenience a top priority. If you have to drive twenty minutes to get there, you're never going to go.

You may find that the best route starts at your front door. A stroll around the neighborhood is fast, easy, and fun. Public parks, running trails, and playgrounds are also great choices. For an indoor workout, check out your local shopping mall. Most malls have plenty of open space, and if you work out early in the day, you may even have the place to yourself.

Once you've found a good location, take the time to scope out some places where you'll be able to feed or change the baby if necessary. A park bench, a children's store, or a shady tree will all work in a pinch. Make sure that your course is well out of the way of car and bicycle traffic, and always be careful when crossing the street with your stroller. Finally, when it comes to working out, variety is key. To keep things interesting, vary the location of your workout.

MOM'S MUSCLES

To maximize the benefits of your workout, you should know something about the muscles you will be training. There are more than six hundred muscles in the human body, and you use all of them. To keep things simple, I'll focus on the muscles Mom uses most. Moving from the feet up, let's learn about the muscles of motherhood:

Gastrocnemius and Soleus (Calf Muscles). These muscles run from your ankles to the backs of your knees. They let you stand on tiptoe when you're try-

Dealing with Injuries

I hate to think about accidents and injuries. But even with the best-designed program, accidents can happen. Here's how to deal with them:

Be prepared. Carry a cell phone and a first-aid kit when you stroll. And sign up for a first-aid or CPR class—you'll learn some helpful tips for dealing with emergencies.

Use the RICE system. The most common injury that may occur after doing Strollercize is a sprained ankle. Whatever the injury, the rule to follow for the first forty-eight hours after an injury is the RICE system:

- Rest/Stop moving the injured area.
- Ice: Ice reduces swelling and helps to ease pain. Put an ice pack on the affected area for 15 to 20 minutes, three or four times a day.
- Compression: Use an Ace bandage, if appropriate, on the injury. Keeping pressure on the injured area will help keep the swelling down.
- Elevation: Elevating the affected limb also helps to reduce swelling.

Get help. If you have fallen, are in a lot of pain, or are bleeding, call for help. Remember, aside from taking care of yourself, you'll need someone to help you care for the baby.

Call your doctor. If the pain is severe, or if the discomfort persists for more than a few hours, have a chat with your doctor to rule out a serious injury.

---

ing to find that last can of formula in the back of the cupboard. They are also used to propel the body forward. And of course, shapely calves look sexy.

Anterior Tibialis. This is the main muscle of your shin, and it runs up the front of your lower leg, from your ankle to your knee. You use this muscle when you tap your toes or activate the brakes on your stroller. It is also a key muscle for jogging, running, and walking. Strengthening and stretching your shins will protect against shin splints (see page 24).

Quadriceps ("Quads"). These four muscles (hence the name) are in the front of your thighs. They allow you to extend your leg, flex your hip, and straighten your knee. They come in handy when you need to get up from the rocking chair while holding your baby, or to lunge down to pick up toys from the floor. Strong quads can also help protect your knees from injury.

Hamstrings. These muscles are in the backs of the thighs. They help bend your knees, extend your thighs, and propel your body forward when you stroll. Your hamstrings tend to get tight during pregnancy, which can limit your movement and put stress on your lower back. Your Strollercize work out will focus on lengthening and strengthening these muscles.

Iliopsoas (Psoas). This muscle is an important member of the **hip flexor** muscle group. It is found in the "diaper area" and runs from the front of each hip, through your pelvis, to your lumbar spine. The psoas muscle stabilizes your pelvis and is a key muscle in proper body alignment. Like the hamstrings, it tends to get shorter and tighter during pregnancy. This can cause lower back pain and hip tightness.

Gluteus Maximus ("Glutes"; Your Butt). This is one of the largest muscles in your body (as if you need anyone to tell you that), and it's important when climbing stairs, straightening your leg behind you, and getting up off the sofa. I don't know why, but this area really seems to attract fat, especially during pregnancy. If you want tight buns, you'll have to work hard to tone that gluteus so it does not become too maximus.

Gluteus Medius (Abductor). This muscle is found at the meaty (and that's putting it nicely) area where your hip meets your outer thigh. It works to extend your leg out to the side and stabilize your hips. It also helps your gluteus maximus rotate your hips outward. This muscle is essential for strolling, while toning the hip area has obvious aesthetic advantages.

Adductors. You may be surprised to learn that there are actually muscles hiding under that jiggly stuff on your inner thighs. The adductor muscles start at your knee and run up the inside of your leg to your pubic bone. These muscles help you to cross your legs when you're wearing that sexy black dress. They also help bring your legs back to the center of your body, to control that postpartum waddle. Many moms use their adductors as kind of a third hand, holding stray objects between their legs. This is actually a great toning move, and I probably don't need to tell you the advantages of having toned inner thighs.

Wrist and Forearm Muscles. Thumbs up or thumbs down? Either way, your forearm muscles get the job done. These muscles run from your wrists up to your elbows, and they are essential for holding and cuddling your baby, as well as for opening the baby's bottle and grasping onto your stroller. Training these muscles will also help you avoid common injuries like carpal tunnel syndrome and tennis elbow.

Biceps. These muscles are found on the fronts of your upper arms. They flex the elbow joint. The Strollercize routine does not target these muscles. Your biceps already get plenty of exercise.

Triceps. These are the muscles on the backs of the upper arms (often thought of as the flabby stuff). Triceps act to extend the arm at the elbow joint, and they tend to be weak, weak, weak. Working these muscles has obvious aesthetic advantages, but strong triceps also come in handy in real-life situations, like getting that stroller up and over a stubborn curb.

Pectorals. Pectorals are your chest muscles. They help move your shoulders and are used to push things—like your stroller. Toned pecs can alleviate upper back pain and give your breasts a more "perky" appearance.

Deltoids ("Delts"). This group of three shoulder muscles—anterior (front), medial (middle), and posterior (back)—are used to raise your arms. Most women have extremely weak delts, which is unfortunate because weak delts can lead to painful shoulder injuries. Strengthening these muscles comes in handy when lifting and carrying heavy objects. Plus, your nice toned delts will look great in that new sleeveless dress.

Rotator Cuff. This group of four small muscles underneath your delts helps keep the shoulder socket intact, which is obviously a good thing. These dainty but powerful muscles need your respect because they are easily injured in everyday activities, from getting your stroller through a doorway to putting the baby in a car seat.

Trapezius ("Traps"). This kite-shaped muscle runs from the nape of your neck, to both shoulders, and down your back to the middle. This is Mom's most overused muscle! By the end of the day, those tired traps are bound to give you some serious shoulder and neck pain. That's why it's important to train this muscle to relax.

Latissimus Dorsi ("Lats"). This key back muscle helps rotate your shoulders. It comes in handy when backing your stroller through doorways, reaching into the cupboard, and changing the sheets of the crib. Strong lats also help you to maintain good posture.

Rhomboids. This small, rectangular-shaped muscle group is found in the center of your back, beneath the hook on your bra. Your rhomboids help you to pull your shoulder blades back so that you can maintain good posture, and they keep your breasts from sagging. Strong rhomboids will counteract that "hunched back" look that is so common in new mothers. That's why breast-feeding moms really need to strengthen and stretch these muscles.

Erector Spinae. These muscles run up from your lower back, up the spine, to the middle of your back. Thanks to your erector spinae, your trunk can twist, turn and bend, movements you make in countless everyday activities. Strengthening these muscles will improve your posture and help fight lower back pain. They also come in handy in "Finding Your Waistline" (see Chapter 8).

Quadratus Lumborum. This is the main lower back muscle that is used to lift the baby from the floor, put her in the crib, or take her out of the stroller. It also helps secure the rib cage during breathing.

Abdominals ("Abs"; the Belly). The abdominals are composed of three main muscles: The **rectus abdominus,** the most exterior of these muscles, runs up the middle front of the torso and is used to bend forward. The **external obliques** and **internal obliques** run diagonally down the sides of the rector abdominus (the external obliques are on top of the internal obliques). They allow you to twist and bend your torso.

Transverse Abdominus. This important muscle is found underneath the other abdominal muscles. It runs from the back of your rib cage to the top of your pelvis and wraps across and all the way around your abdomen, like a corset. The transverse abdominus works to pull the other muscles toward your trunk and to stabilize your spine. Of all your abdominal muscles, the transverse is the most heavily involved in childbirth. Training this muscle is key to slimming your post-partum waistline. The abdominal muscles affect many parts of the body and can prevent a lot of injuries. In particular, they support the lower back.

Pelvic Floor (Kegel Muscles). The muscles of the pelvic floor form a figure eight around the anus, vagina, and urethra. These muscles not only support the contents of your pelvis (i.e., the uterus, bladder, and bowel), but also control bowel and bladder activity and aid in sexual pleasure. The pelvic floor takes a lot of pressure during pregnancy and childbirth. So if you ever want to be able to "hold it" again (see Chapter 5), you'd better start training your pelvic floor.

SAFETY CHECK

Last but not least is your safety. For safe strolling, always take the following precautions:

- **Consult your doctor before beginning this or any other exercise program.**

- **Never leave your child unattended in the stroller.** It takes only a few seconds for an accident to happen, so don't turn your back for a moment. To avoid a runaway stroller, keep at least one hand on the stroller at all times. When parking on an incline, turn your stroller sideways. And if you need your hands free, lock the wheels of the stroller.

- **Drive a safe stroller.** Follow the tips in Chapter 3 for selecting a safe and durable stroller. And know how to use it.

- **Always strap the baby into the stroller, and make sure that the straps fit snugly.** Never rely on just the safety bar, because the baby can slip out underneath. Check frequently to be sure the straps stay tight and secure. (Some older babies can learn how to loosen or even release the restraints.)

- **Always stroll on a smooth surface.** That way you can avoid too much vibration and jarring for the baby. Keep a lookout for sticks, cracks, gutters, potholes, and curbs. Avoid strolling on ice or mud or through big puddles. Not only could you slip and lose your balance, but you will rust out the stroller's wheels.

- **Avoid hanging bags or other objects from the handlebar.** The stroller can become unbalanced and tip over. You should avoid blankets that can get caught in the wheels of the stroller. Instead, use blankets that are specially designed to be attached, securely, to the stroller.

- **Wear bright colors.** That way you can be seen by automobile and bicycle traffic. Remember, dark-colored strollers are difficult to see. Avoid exercising at dawn or dusk or at any other time when visibility is reduced. For added safety, wear reflective clothing, and put reflectors on your stroller (available at sporting goods and bicycle shops).

- **Keep your eyes on the road.** Look both ways when you cross the street. And never put the stroller in the street while you are waiting at an intersection. If you're strolling with a partner, avoid heavy discussions that may distract you from safe strolling.

- **Never Strollercize on an empty stomach.** Have a light snack one hour before working out. Drink fluids before, during, and after your workout, and be on the lookout for signs of dehydration (see page 37).

- **Avoid exercising to the point of exhaustion.** You need to keep your mind clear and focused to care for your baby.

- **Dress yourself and the baby appropriately for the weather.** Remember, since you'll be the one moving, you will probably feel warmer than the baby. If the weather is iffy, bring a rain shield for the stroller, just to be safe.

- **Do not stroll alone in isolated areas.** Always tell someone where and when you are going to stroll. And if possible, stroll with a buddy.

- **Bring your first-aid kit and a cell phone (if you have one) in case of an emergency.**

- **Stop exercising if you feel dizzy, nauseous, faint, or short of breath or if any of the moves become painful.** See your doctor if these symptoms persist.

Now that you know the basics, you're ready to start Strollercizing. So what are you waiting for?

.... *5* ....

Your Waist Away

*N*obody needs to tell you that your waistline took a beating during pregnancy. Just glance down, and you'll see the damage. After nine months of stretching in ways you could never have imagined possible, suddenly that big beach ball of a tummy deflates, and you're left with a mid-section that's saggy, flabby, and numb.

After the birth of my third child, Romeu, people told me that I had better get used to my new fleshy belly. After all, one pregnancy is bad enough, but three strikes and you're out. Of course, I didn't listen. Instead, I created a complete abdominal routine, capable of toning up even the flabbiest of bellies (including my own). This chapter introduces the Strollercize abdominal and waistline routine, called Waist Away. I have also included a series of pelvic floor exercises that are a must to do before you start your abdominal routine. Follow this plan, and I guarantee that you'll be wearing that bathing suit in no time.

HOLDING IT!

The birth of my second child, Lorenzo, taught me the true meaning of being in "control." In those first few postpartum weeks, I was afraid to laugh, sneeze, or jog, as "holding it" had become utterly impossible. I was humbled and humiliated when I lost control of my bladder while strolling down Fifth Avenue. The saddest part was that I was too embarrassed to tell anyone. I thought that sort of thing only happened to "old women." Over the years, I've heard more and more Strollercize moms share similar stories. And I've come to realize that postpartum incontinence is actually a very common condition. That's why I designed the following routine: to help new moms regain control.

The secret to "holding it" is to strengthen the muscles of the pelvic floor. These important muscles are found at the base of the pelvis, where they work to support the pelvic organs and control urination and defecation. Ideally, the pelvic floor muscles should be nice and tight. But during pregnancy the increased weight of the fetus and the uterus, as well as increased levels of the hormone progesterone, can cause them to stretch, sag, and weaken. Postpartum, even simple movements like lifting the baby, laughing, or coughing can stress these muscles, causing a mom to lose control. And don't even think about doing any strenuous exercise without training these muscles. Not only will you risk wet undies, but you could make this condition worse.

Whether you're leaking or not, it's important to train your pelvic floor muscles because it will strengthen your abdominals too! The majority of women suffer some pelvic floor damage during pregnancy—with or without symptoms. Besides, strengthening your pelvic floor will improve your sex life and help you get that nice flat tummy. For best results, start these exercises as soon after delivery as possible. You should do each move at least once a day (the more often, the better). The entire routine takes about five minutes. Each exercise targets a different spot in the pelvic floor area. Many of the exercises can be done anywhere, even in your hospital bed. Just be sure to empty the contents of your bladder before you begin—we don't want any accidents!

Finding Your Pelvic Floor

For many moms, the pelvic floor muscles are so out of shape that it's hard to tell if they're using them. So before you can start strengthening these muscles, you'll have to find them. This move will help you get back in touch with your pelvic floor.

1. To best feel your PF muscles at work, sit with your knees bent in front of you and your heels under your buttocks, as if you were dining in a Japanese restaurant. (Note: If this is too intense for your knees, shift to the side and rest your buns on the ground.)

2. Relax your bottom and all of the muscles of the entire pelvic floor area.

3. After you have relaxed these muscles completely, slowly begin to tighten them. Imagine that you are pulling on the drawstring of a laundry bag, as you pull your pelvic floor high up into your body. Slowly pull the laundry bag closed—the slower the better. You may feel that you can't tighten anymore, but keep trying. If you are doing this right, you should feel a shaking sensation in the pelvic floor region.

4. Hold for 20 counts (or longer if you can).

5. Now slowly relax and let the muscles go loose again.

Repeat 10 to 20 times.

$\cdots$

At first it may be difficult to contract your PF muscles without contracting your abdominal and buttocks muscles. Keep trying. You'll get much better results from your pelvic floor routine. You can use your hands to help you focus on the PF contraction. Make a tight fist when you are contracting your PF muscles (but keep the rest of your body relaxed). Then relax your hand as you relax the muscles.

Tighten and Loosen

Now that you've found your pelvic floor, it's time to really shake things up.

1. Start in the Finding Your Pelvic Floor position (remember the Japanese restaurant).

2. Contract and lift your PF muscles until they start to shake.

3. Hold this position for 20 seconds. You should feel more than a tremor.

4. Slowly lower the pelvic floor, but only halfway. Take a brief rest.

5. Tighten your muscles again as much as you can, and bring the pelvic floor back up until you shake.

Do 10 to 20 reps.

· · · · ·

You can do this exercise in almost any position, but this is the best way to feel your PF muscles at work.

Isolations

Your body is a complex system in which everything is connected. Normally, your PF muscles work together with your lower abs and glutes. This simple move will help you isolate your PF muscles.

1. Start by positioning yourself on your hands and knees.

2. Lower your head to the floor. Your hands and arms should be directly under your shoulders, and your knees should be under your hips.

3. Completely relax your pelvic floor. If you're doing this right, your butt will stick out and your tummy will bulge a bit.

4. Now slowly contract the pelvic floor, leaving your buttocks and abdominals loose. Get as deep into your body as possible, focusing on tightening your urethra rather than just the vaginal area. Remember, your goal is to isolate those PF muscles. No other part of your body should move.

Repeat 10 times.

Ball Game

This is another great move for your pelvic floor. You can do this exercise anywhere, even while watching a ball game.

1. Sit on the edge of a sturdy chair, couch, or bleacher. Keep your feet under your knees, your knees bent, and your legs wide apart.

2. Rest your elbows on your knees, and imagine that you are holding a soft ball in your hands.

3. Let your body get completely limp and relaxed. Your belly will bulge, and your pelvic floor should melt into the seat of the chair or sofa.

4. Now contract your PF muscles, and lift them high off the seat. Your buns should be relaxed and still glued to the seat.

5. Squeeze that imaginary ball in your hands to help you focus on the PF contraction. And don't forget to breathe.

6. Hold for 20 seconds and release.

Repeat 10 times.

Gotta Go's

This move is based on what you probably do when you've really gotta go but there's no bathroom in sight. Actually, crossing your legs is one of the most difficult positions from which to control your bladder. But it's a great position for working those PF muscles.

1. Stand with one leg crossed in front of the other and your hands on your buttocks. Keep your chest lifted, and look up at the sky.

2. Contract your PF muscles, and squeeze them without squeezing your legs or buttocks.

3. Hold for 20 seconds and release.

Repeat 10 times.

Sleep Tight

Just because you're lying down in this exercise doesn't mean you're getting a break. In fact, this is probably the most advanced move of the bunch. It may take a while to get the hang of it, but once you've mastered it, you can be sure that your pelvic floor is in tip-top shape.

1. Lie on your side, with your knees bent and your top hand sandwiched between your thighs.

2. Tighten your PF muscles, without squeezing your inner thighs and buns. Hold this position until you shake.

3. Now try to hold the contraction in your pelvic floor as you try to relax your buttocks muscles as much as you can. This may seem impossible at first, but don't give up. You'll get a grip on it!

Now that your pelvic floor is toned and tightened, let's work up to the real loose stuff—your waist—and let's get it toned and tightened too.

THE EARLY WEEKS

The only way to get your abs back is through serious exercise. But you have to start slowly. Remember, your muscles are weak. In the early weeks, getting up out of bed should be your most strenuous abdominal activity. And if you have a diastasis, you'll need to be even more careful. Some experts believe that abdominal exercises like sit-ups and crunches can worsen the separation of the abdominal muscles. The Strollercize routine does not include these moves. But you should still play it safe and go easy on your abs until your diastasis has healed. The following exercise will help to close the gap and correct this condition.

Testing for Diastasis Recti

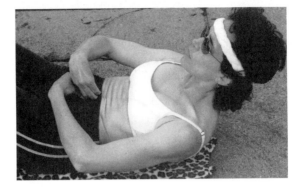

As we discussed in Chapter 1, for some new moms, the rectus abdominus muscles stretch so much during pregnancy that the two sides, or recti, start to separate. This condition is called diastasis recti. You should test for a diastasis before you begin your Strollercize abdominal routine, and modify your workout accordingly.

Lie on your back with your knees bent and your feet flat on the floor. Place the fingertips of one hand firmly into the belly button area. See if you can feel the ridges of muscle on either side of your fingers. Now gently lift your head up about eight inches off the floor. If your fingers fall into a gap, then you have a diastasis. The bigger the gap (i.e., the more fingers you can fit inside), the worse the condition. A one-inch or two-inch gap is nothing to worry about. A diastasis is only a problem if the gap is three or four inches wide (i.e., if you can fit three or four fingers in the gap). If you think you have diastasis recti, you should confirm it with your doctor.

The Baby's Up

I call this exercise The Baby's Up because it mimics the movement you do when you get up in the middle of the night to check on the baby. I have three kids, so I practice this move a lot.

1. Lie on your back with your knees up and your feet about 8 inches from your bottom.

2. Put your hands around your waistline and pull it in, as if you were closing the seam of a ripped shirt.

3. Now lift your head up and exhale, just as you do when you are getting up for the baby. Hold for 5 counts, and bring the abdominal muscles in tight, as if you were cinching a corset.

4. As you lower your head, try to maintain the contraction in the abs. Inhale when your head touches the floor, but don't relax your tummy muscles.

Do 20 repetitions. Repeat this exercise 3 times a day.

•••••

Diastasis or not, Strollercize recommends that you wait six weeks before launching into the full-blown abdominal routine (possibly longer if you've had a C-section and are still feeling uncomfortable). Until then, stick with simple moves like The Baby's Up, Finding Your Waistline—Lying Down (page 75), and Make It Go Away (page 76). These exercises are also safe to do if you have a diastasis. And you should start working your pelvic floor muscles as soon as possible!

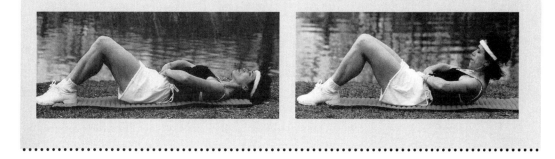

Training Tips

Here are some tips for getting the most out of your Strollercize abdominal routine:

- *Don't hold your breath. Think about pulling in—not sucking in—so you'll remember to keep breathing while contracting your abdominals.*

- *Exhale on the exertion (i.e., the hard part), and avoid breathing into your belly. Many people have the tendency to push out their abs when they're exerting themselves. But this sort of belly breathing trains your muscles the wrong way and can lead to a poochy abdomen.*

- *Always start your routine by Finding Your Waistline—Lying Down (see page 75). This move will elongate your spine and help you get in touch with your midsection. Return to this move frequently throughout your routine to give your back and abdominals a rest.*

- *Remember, your abdominal muscles wrap all the way around your torso. Many of the moves in your Strollercize Waist Away routine target the lower back muscles. You may feel tight in this area, so take it easy until you get stronger.*

- *If you feel continued pain or stiffness, stop the exercise and consult your doctor.*

- *Some of the most effective abdominal moves are also very subtle. If you're not feeling the effects of a particular move, check your form and try again. A sensation of warmth or vibration in your midsection is a positive sign that you're targeting the right muscles.*

- *If you had a C-section, go easy on your abdominal routine until you regain your strength.*

THE WAIST WORK

The following exercises will increase your muscle tone, improve your posture, and help you to reconnect with your abdominal muscles. For best results, do your waistline routine every day. All you need is an open space, the family room floor, the backyard—almost anywhere will do. Just be sure you have enough room to lie down and stretch out your arms. If you're not comfortable on the bare floor, grab an exercise mat or a baby blanket. If the baby's awake, you can put him next to you in his bouncy seat, and he can be your personal trainer.

Finding Your Waistline—Lying Down

If finding your waistline sounds easy, just look in the mirror. If you're like most new moms, all that you'll find is a fleshy deposit of skin and fat where your waist used to be. An essential part of reclaiming your waistline is remembering where it is. This move will help.

1. Start by lying on your back with your knees bent and your feet about twelve inches from your buttocks. Keep your chin lifted, your chest up, and your neck relaxed. Try to maintain the natural curve in your spine. (If you're doing this right, your partner should be able to slide a pencil under the small of your back.) Place your fingers around your midsection, where your waist used to be. Close your eyes, and visualize that teeny, tiny waist.

2. Now pull in your tummy, and see if you can make a belt with your fingers. Imagine that you are buttoning your navel to your uterus. Take a minute to pull in at the waist and get in touch with the muscular energy in your abdomen.

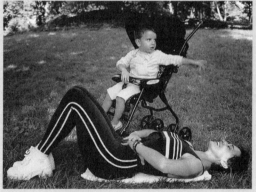

This Finding Your Waistline experience should take about 30 seconds.

Come back to this exercise between the tougher abdominal exercises to release tension in the lower back.

Make It Go Away

You see all the gunk that's been collecting around your waistline? Well, this move will make it go away!

1. Sit up straight with your knees bent and your feet about 2 feet from your buttocks. Grab hold of your knees—or the hands of your baby!

2. Slowly round your back, and begin to lower your upper body toward the floor.

3. When you are halfway there, stop and wave your hands in the air as if to magically make your tummy disappear. If you're doing this right, you'll feel a shaking sensation in the middle of the abdominals. Hold this position for 10 counts.

4. Sit back up again, Find Your Waistline, and give your back a rest.

As you get stronger you will be able to hold the position for 30 counts or more. Aim for 3 sets.

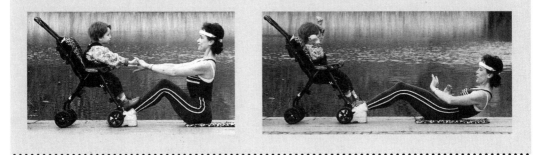

The Diaper

Believe it or not, the diaper change is a great workout for your baby. Every time you lift up those tiny toes, the baby is getting a delicious stretch in the lower spine and a gentle crunch in those tiny abs. Now it's your turn to be the baby (only no one's going to help you lift up that hefty behind).

1. Lie on your back with your knees bent and your heels resting on your buttocks. Keep your chin lifted, your eyes looking up, and your neck relaxed.

2. Reach your arms over your head, and grab hold of a sturdy object like the leg of a bed, a piano, or your stroller.

3. Try to bring your knees to your chest as you lift your butt off the floor, as if someone could slip a diaper underneath.

4. Keep your head on the floor as you pull in your abs and bring your knees even closer to your chest.

5. Lower slowly to the ground.

Start by doing 10 of these little crunches, then work up to 20. If you'd like, you can do a few sets, but be sure you rest in between by Finding Your Waistline.

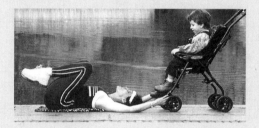 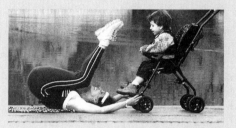

Swipes

This simple variation on the Diaper targets the sides of your waist. During this exercise, try to visualize the way you clean and swipe your baby's bottom.

1. Bring your knees up toward your chest, just as you did for the Diaper. You may cross your feet at the ankles.

2. Now twist your knees to the right, and let your feet move left. Again, hold on to a sturdy object. Try to get your butt off the floor to fully contract and recruit your obliques.

Do 10 reps, then switch sides.

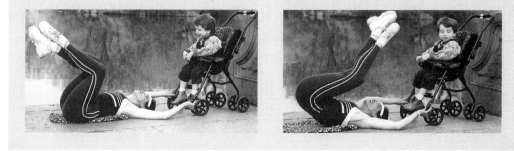

Changing

Ask any mom what she would most like to change about her body, and chances are she'll point to her waistline. This exercise will help.

1. Lie on your back with your knees bent and your feet about 12 inches from your buttocks.

2. Find Your Waistline.

3. Stretch your arms over your head, and grab hold of your stroller (or another sturdy object).

4. Slowly bend your knees, and bring them close to your chest. If necessary, use your hands to pull your knees up.

5. Hold for several seconds.

6. Now keep your knees together and slowly lower your legs to the right side of your body.

7. Bring your knees back to center, and repeat on the left side.

Do 10 to 20 repetitions on each side. This exercise will get the twist back into your torso and wake up your obliques.

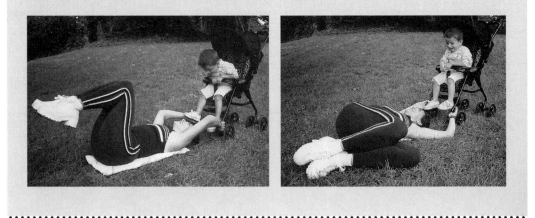

Painting the Ceiling

This exercise will stretch your hamstrings and work your lower abs. It may also come in handy if you haven't finished painting the nursery.

1. Lie on your back with your knees bent.

2. Find Your Waistline.

3. Reach your arms over your head, and grab onto a sturdy object.

4. Now raise your right leg up into the air, keeping your foot flexed. Try to get your foot in line with your waistline. Pretend you have baby blue paint on the sole of your right foot.

5. Now lift your left leg up, and pretend that this foot has pink paint.

6. Slowly exchange your legs in the air, and imagine that you are painting the ceiling as you stretch your legs.

Do 10 to 20 cycles.

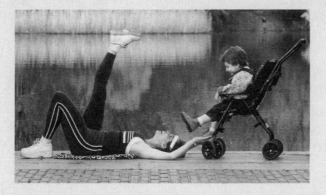

This exercise will be tough at first because your hamstrings are probably tight. Keep trying! It will lengthen your hamstrings and lower back, while toning your belly.

Forevers

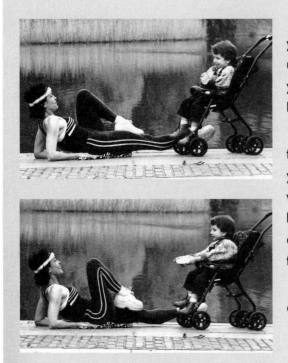

1. Start by lying on your back with your elbows bent and your hands under your lower back. Imagine that you are relaxing on the beach in a tiny bikini.

2. Stretch your right leg out in front of you, touching the ground. Bring your left knee up toward your chest, with your foot pointing toward your butt. Keep your toes pointed. If you're doing this right, your legs should form a figure 4.

3. Now switch legs, keeping your chin lifted and your abs pulled in tight.

Do 10 to 20 reps.

• • • • •

Note: This advanced exercise really works the lower abs. If you just had a C-section, be sure to take it easy.

Side Get-Ups

How many times do you get out of bed at night to tend to your baby? Well, here's a chance to turn all of those late-night trips to the nursery into a serious abdominal workout. This move will tone up your waistline, and if you need to get up twenty times during the night—you'll be ready.

1. Lie down on your left side, with your left arm tucked under your head for support. Your left leg is bent, and your right leg is relaxed and long, as if you were "spooning" next to your partner. Let your right arm drape across your chest. Pretend that you're fast asleep, but don't get too comfortable—any minute now the baby will be calling you.

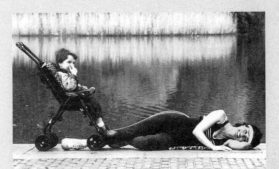

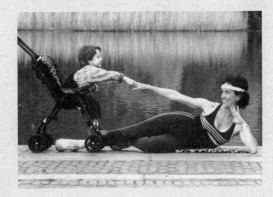

2. When you're ready to rise, stretch your right arm out over your right leg and use the momentum to lift your torso up. Keep your left elbow on the ground to support the crunch. Try to keep your lower body on the ground, and focus the work on your oblique muscles, along the side of your waist. You should feel the contraction in your obliques.

3. Hold for a few seconds, then slowly lower down to the starting position.

Do 5 to 20 reps on each side. When you are stronger, you can try to do this exercise without the support of the elbow.

• • • • •

(In the photo, I'm holding the position by reaching for my son's hand. If your child is old enough to participate like this, I encourage it. Your little "coach" will keep you motivated!)

Where's Mommy?

I watched all of my children do this beautiful move. Then one day I realized the benefits this exercise could have on my own waistline. So far we've focused on the front of the torso. This move balances things out by focusing on your backside. It also targets that dreaded back fat (i.e., the fleshy stuff behind the hips).

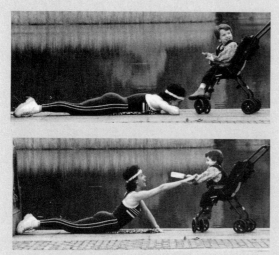

1. Lie on your tummy, with your hands underneath your chin and your elbows out to the side. Tighten your butt, and pull in your abs.

2. Now slowly lift your chest off the floor, using your left hand for support as your right hand reaches up into the air. Go as high as you can.

3. Hold for a second, then lower and switch hands.

Work up to 10 reps.

• • • • •

At first your back may be tight, and you won't be able to lift up very high. But after a few weeks, you should be able to do this exercise with both hands in the air.

Good work, Mom! You have just completed the Strollercize Waist Away workout. How about giving yourself a pat on that nice firm belly! Remember, for best results, you should do this routine every day. After a few weeks, you'll be ready to move on to the complete Strollercize workout. But you'll still need your daily dose of abs.

II

Your Strollercize Workout

. . . .

The following chapters introduce the Strollercize workout. This routine will give you a total-body workout, targeting the areas that you need to work the most. Chapters 6 and 7 present, respectively, the warm-up and aerobic components of your workout. Chapter 8 focuses on strengthening all of the major muscle groups in your body. Finally, Chapter 9 introduces a series of stretches that will help you relax, prevent injuries, and seal in the benefits of your workout.

For best results, I recommend that you do the entire routine from start to finish at least twice a week, and add the Strollercize Waist Away routine (Chapter 5) every day. Once you get the hang of it, you'll be able to complete the entire workout in less than an hour. That breaks down to about 20 to 30 minutes of cardiovascular activity and 15 to 20 minutes of upper- and lower-body conditioning and stretching, plus ab work. If you don't have time to do the entire routine, you can do your aerobic and conditioning workouts on different days. Just be sure to warm up before each workout and cool down after.

................6................

Warming Up

By the time you dress the baby, pack the diaper bag, and maneuver the stroller through your front door (and I hope you don't have too many porch steps), chances are you're already huffing and puffing. Getting out of the house with the baby is already a serious warm-up. Still, it's always a good idea to take a few minutes to focus your mind and get in touch with your muscles before you start Strollercizing.

Warming up is essential for preventing injuries. If you're not already sweating by the time you've made it out the door (or if you're staying indoors), start your warm-up with five to ten minutes of gentle aerobic activity, like taking a brisk walk or marching in place. Your goal is to break a light sweat and get your heart rate moderately elevated. Next it's time to wake up those muscles. The following moves should do the trick. Don't forget to lock the wheels of the stroller before you start.

Toddler Watch

This move warms up the muscles in your neck—and will help you keep track of your wandering toddler in the years to come.

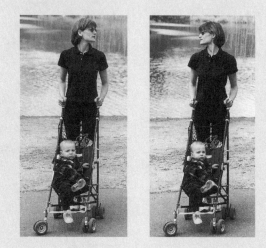

1. Start in your Strollercize posture check position, with both hands on the stroller.

2. Turn your head to the right as far as you can. Your chin should be in line with the seam of your shirt.

3. Now turn your head to the left.

4. Repeat on both sides until you've gotten the kinks out of your neck.

Wipies

Imagine that your happy toddler has just created his very first Crayon masterpiece—on your living-room wall. This move will help you clean up the mess, while opening up your shoulders.

1. Start by standing tall, with your right hand on the stroller. Your knees should be slightly bent, and your buns slightly out—not tucked.

2. Extend your left arm out to the side, and flex your wrist.

3. Circle your arm backward as if you were wiping a wall. You should feel the stretch in your shoulders and chest.

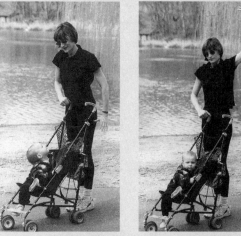

Do about 5 circles on each side, or until you feel the range of motion increase and your shoulder starts to feels warm.

· · · · ·

The shoulder joints are easily injured, so be very careful and deliberate as you wipe.

Stroll Aways

This move opens up the waist, back, and spine. It may even help roll away the unwanted flesh that is collecting around your midsection. You'll need to unlock the wheels of the stroller before you begin.

1. Stand with your right hip facing the stroller and your knees slightly bent.
2. Place your right hand on the handlebar, and your left hand on your waist.
3. Take a deep breath.
4. On the exhale, bend to the right at your waist, extend your right arm, and push the stroller away from your body. All of the movement should be in your upper body. Be sure that your legs are in the Strollercize posture check position with your heels firmly planted on the ground. Keep your knees slightly soft to accommodate the movement.
5. Imagine your new, beautifully elongated waistline as you feel the stretch on the left side of your waist.
6. Repeat on the left side.

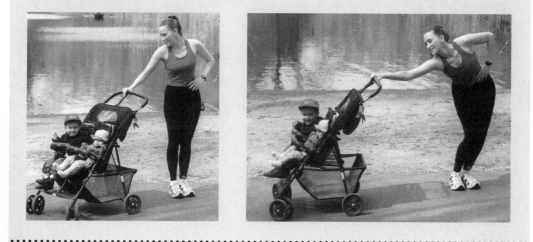

Bubble Gum

When you step in something sticky (and it happens to the best of us), this is a great way to assess the damage. This move also stretches your thigh muscles.

1. Stand with your right hand on the stroller, your feet under your hips, and your knees slightly bent.

2. Bring the heel of your left foot up behind your body. (If necessary, you can use your left hand to grab your foot.)

3. Now turn your head and look over your left shoulder to check out the bottom of your shoe.

4. Assuming that your shoe is gum free, grasp the arch of the left foot with your left hand and stick your heel into your left bun.

5. Hold this position for a few seconds.

6. Check out your other shoe.

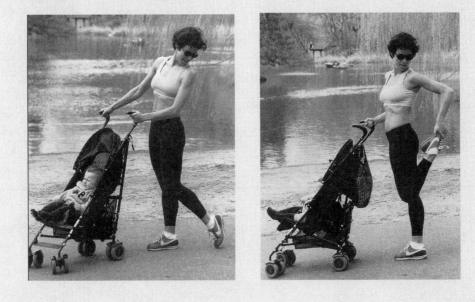

The Counter

Have you ever climbed up onto the kitchen counter to dig out that lost box of cookies? Well, then you probably felt a great stretch in your hips, thighs, and buttocks.

1. Hold the stroller with your left hand. Shift your weight onto your left leg, and keep your left knee soft. (Don't "lock" the joint in a straight position.)

2. Lift your right leg sideways from your hip, and grab hold of your knee with your right hand. Try to keep your chest up. To get the full benefits of this stretch, you must lift your ankle to the same height as your knee.

3. Repeat on the right.

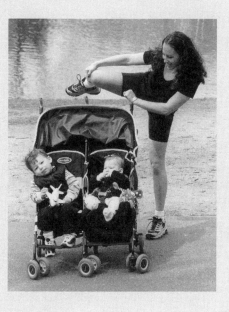

Peek-a-Boo

This is a great way to entertain your baby while warming up your inner thighs.

1. Stand behind the stroller, with your toes pointing straight ahead. Hold on to the stroller for support.

2. Now widen your stance until your feet are about 4 feet apart.

3. Sit back, bend your knees, and get as low as you can as you gently bend forward at the hip. Keep the weight of your body on your heels.

4. Now glide to the right, putting all of your body weight on your right leg. Your left leg should be stretched to the side.

5. Say "peek-a-boo" to the baby.

6. Glide toward the left side of the stroller.

• • • • •

If the baby giggles and squeals, you'll know you're doing it right.

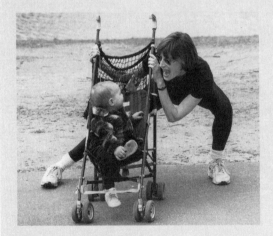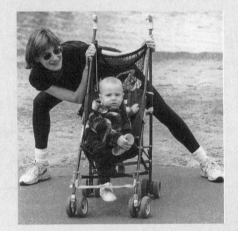

The Brakes

You'll do this move at least 20 times a day, whenever you activate the brakes on the stroller. But it's also a great way to warm up the ankles and shins.

1. Stand behind your stroller, with your right hand on the handlebar.

2. Shift your weight onto your right leg, and flex your left foot out, directly in front of your left hip. Keep your chest lifted and your elbow out. Your buttocks should be neutral, not tucked under your body. Remember to keep your abdominals pulled up and tight.

3. Now point and flex your left foot, until you feel the warmth in your shin. Your left leg should be straight, and the heel should touch the ground between flexes.

4. Repeat on the other side.

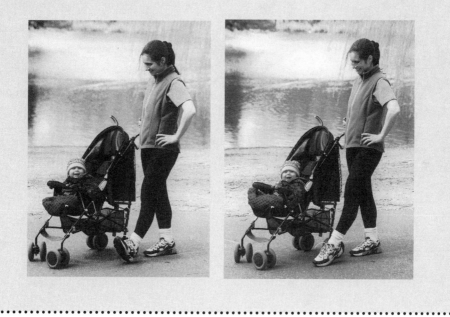

Shoelaces

Remember the end of your pregnancy, when you couldn't bend over to lace your shoes? Now is the time to celebrate your newly discovered freedom and flexibility.

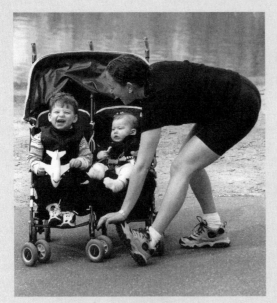

1. Start in the Brakes position, with your right hand on the stroller, your left leg extended, and your toes pointing toward the sky.

2. Stick your buns out behind you as you bend forward from the hip.

3. Now reach for your shoelaces with your left wrist (or your socks, or your shins, depending on how flexible you are). If you are very flexible, you'll be able to kiss your knees. Try to keep your back flat, with most of your body weight on your right leg, and keep your front leg as straight as possible.

4. Stay in this position for 10 seconds—until you can reach those laces!

5. Repeat on the right side.

High Heels

If you fondly remember the old days of tight dresses and high heels, this move is for you. Sure, those high heels made your legs look super sexy. But try wearing them to the playground. This exercise will wake up the muscles of the lower legs and will give them that high-heeled look—no matter what kind of shoes you're wearing.

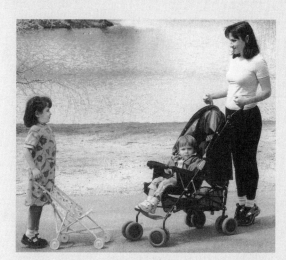

1. Hold on to the stroller with both hands, and find your Strollercize posture.

2. With your anklebones together, slowly rise onto the balls of your feet. Imagine that you're wearing a sexy pair of stilettos.

3. Now lower your heels to the ground, and rise back up again. Repeat 5 times.

4. On your fifth repetition, squeeze your legs together, contract your butt, abs tight, and balance in the "high-heeled" position for 10 seconds.

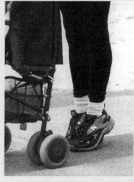

Good job! You've completed your warm-up. You should feel focused, loose, and ready to Strollercize!

The Heart of the Matter

*W*elcome to the aerobic component of your Strollercize workout. This is your chance to work up a sweat, burn some fat, and condition your cardiovascular system. For maximum benefits, you should do the Strollercize aerobic routine at least twice a week to get the fitness benefits. Aim for a minimum of twenty to thirty minutes of continuous strolling, working at 65 to 80 percent of your maximum heart rate (see below). Start with a duration and intensity that feels comfortable to you, and increase gradually as you feel ready. And remember to pace yourself. If you start to feel tired or dizzy, slow down to a more comfortable place. Always do your warm-up before you begin your aerobic routine. And once you get going, avoid stopping suddenly if your heart rate is up. If you need to tend to the baby, try marching in place—but don't stop moving your legs.

MEASURING YOUR HEART RATE

The best way to tell if you're working hard enough to achieve your goals is to measure your heart rate (i.e., the number of times your heart beats per minute). The idea is to challenge your heart to work harder, but not too hard. Strollercize recommends that you aim for 70 to 80 percent of your *maximum heart rate* (i.e., the maximum number of times that your heart can beat in a minute). This *target heart rate* (THR) will be different for each person, depending on your age and fitness level.

To calculate your target heart rate, first find your maximum heart rate. Start with the number 220 (i.e., the maximum heart rate at birth), and subtract your age.

So if you're 32 years old, 220 − 32 = 188. Your maximum heart rate is 188.

Next, take your maximum heart rate, and multiply it by the percentage at which you want to train (i.e., 70 to 80 percent). The result will be your target heart rate.

Suppose you want to train at 70 percent of your maximum heart rate. 188 × 0.70 = 131. Your target heart rate is 131 beats per minute.

Finally, to figure out your heart rate for a 10-second count (see below), divide your target heart rate by 6.

131 ÷ 6 = 21. Your target heart rate for a 10-second count is 21.

To measure your heart rate, place your index and middle fingers along the side of your neck, in the natural groove. Don't press too hard. You'll know when you've found the right place because you'll feel your heartbeat thumping. Now look at your watch, and count the number of beats, starting at zero, for 10 seconds. Calculate your target heart rate (see above), or use the chart below to find out if you're in your target training zone.

TARGET HEART RATE ZONE
(for a 10 second count)

| Your Age | *Percent of Maximum Heart Rate* | | | | | | |
	55%	60%	65%	70%	75%	80%	85%
20	18	20	22	23	25	27	28
25	18	19	20	22	24	26	27
30	17	18	19	22	23	25	26
35	17	18	19	21	22	24	25
40	17	18	19	20	21	23	24
45	16	17	18	19	20	22	23

Practice checking your heart rate before you start Strollercizing. Once you've gotten the hang of it, you should check your heart rate several times during your cardio workout. Since it is difficult to take your pulse while strolling, you should stop and brake your stroller. But keep your legs marching in place.

THE STROLLS

Each of the following moves targets a different muscle group in your body, and they will all keep your heart rate soaring. For best results, try to maintain a brisk pace (between 3.5 and 4.5 miles an hour, depending on your fitness level). To get an idea of how fast you're strolling, you can measure the length of your route using your car odometer, time how long it takes you to walk a mile on the treadmill, or purchase a pedometer to wear when you stroll.

You should always start your routine with the Basic Stroll. This move will form the backbone of your aerobic workout. Return to this stroll frequently, especially if you need to take a breather. (FYI: This move is also great for everyday strolling.)

The Basic Stroll

The Basic Stroll is all about good posture and a great attitude. Look at the mother in the picture. Not only is she a shining example of perfect stroller form, but her body language says, "I'm proud to be a mom!"

1. When you're strolling with the baby, visualize yourself not as an overworked, overstressed mother, but as a woman who is in control of herself and proud of her beautiful baby. You are strong, you are powerful, and you are going to get a great workout. And don't forget your form: Your chin is up, and your shoulders are down. Your chest should be lifted, with your elbows out and your wrists straight. Try to maintain a firm but relaxed grip on the stroller. Your belly button should be hugging your spine, and don't slouch!

2. As you stroll, your feet should point straight ahead, and your heels should touch the ground before the balls of your feet. Make sure that your feet stay within the wheels of the stroller. Keep your legs under your hips, and don't be afraid to let your thighs rub together.

3. Finally, with each step, try to reach your leg out in front of your belly button. Your steps should be silent and deliberate. Avoid shuffling your feet or dragging your heels. And don't bang your feet down hard on the pavement.

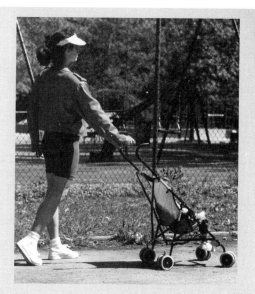

· · · · ·

Once you've mastered the Basic Stroll, you can try some of the variations listed below. You can do the moves in any order, but be sure to vary your routine so you don't get bored or overtire a muscle group.

The Miniskirt Stroll

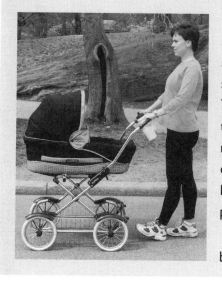

1. For this move, imagine that you're wearing a sexy little miniskirt and you're showing off your stuff. Your tummy is tight, and your thighs are squeezed together (otherwise the skirt won't fit). You have to take very fast, very small steps (in a tight skirt, your legs don't have a lot of room to move around). Keep your perfect posture, and cruise like a vixen. Keep a good grip on the stroller. Let your hips swing from side to side, as fast as possible, in one smooth and continuous motion.

2. Keep up this movement until your buns burn.

Of all the strolls, this one is the best for your butt. To get the full effects, be sure to take this move to its maximum speed and swing velocity. Pretty soon you'll be fitting into that miniskirt.

The Mom-on-a-Mission Stroll

This is no Sunday-afternoon stroll. You're a mom on a mission. It's time to pick up your pace and feel those muscles in motion. This move will stretch out the fronts of the hips while increasing your gluteal power.

1. The key to this move is to take big steps. As you stroll, imagine that your legs are long like a dancer's, and try to extend each leg as far in front of your body as possible without sacrificing your stroller posture. Focus on how good it feels to stretch your legs and how much distance you are covering with each long stride. If you're doing this right, your feet may occasionally hit the wheels of the stroller. Be careful not to stub your toes!

2. Once you've got the hang of it, you can try holding on to the stroller with only your right hand. Move along the left side of the stroller, and take advantage of the extra space. Bring your upper body into the action by swinging your left arm alongside your body.

3. Now try the same thing with your left hand on the stroller.

Be sure to log in equal time on both sides.

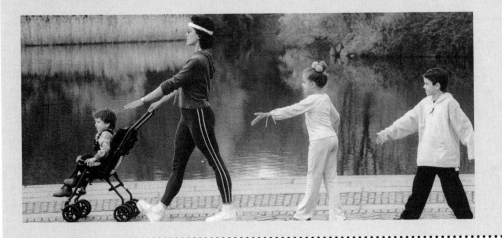

The Rolling Stroll

The baby is crying, the doorbell is ringing, and you're down to your last diaper. Yes, your new life is crazy, and hectic, and dizzying. And I want to bring that same intensity to your workout. Now it's time to really pick up the pace and get your heart rate soaring. Give this move everything you've got, and you'll feel the stresses of life roll away.

1. The Rolling Stroll should give you the feeling of jogging, without all the strain on your body and your stroller. Find a swift pace that feels comfortable for your lower body and legs. Focus on pushing ground behind you as you roll forward. Keep your elbows out and your wrists straight. Your buns and hips should be underneath your shoulders, and don't lean over the stroller. Stay erect.

2. If your breasts are tender, you can try holding on to the stroller with one hand and placing the other arm across your chest to support them. Just be sure to switch arms from time to time.

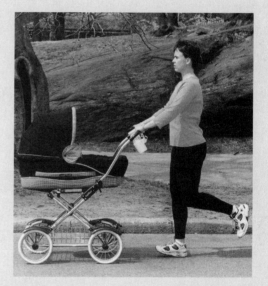

3. Remember that you're moving fast, but you're not running: Your heels should always hit the ground first, and your feet should stay low to the ground. As you stroll, you should feel a strong sensation up the backs of your legs in your hamstring muscles.

· · · · ·

I tell my Strollercize moms to pace themselves when strolling. When you start to feel tired, switch to a different stroll to give your leg muscles a break and your heart rate a chance to recover. As your fitness level increases, you should be able to perform this aerobic roll for longer periods of time.

The Galloping Gal

For this stroll, imagine that you're galloping into the sunset on a big, black stallion. This exercise focuses on the hips and gives your shins and calves a break.

1. With your right hand on the stroller, turn so that your right hip is next to the stroller.

2. Take long, sideways steps, looking over your right shoulder so you can see where you're going. Bend forward slightly at the hips, and stick your buns out behind you. And don't be afraid to let those thighs slap together as you go.

3. Switch sides, and enjoy the ride.

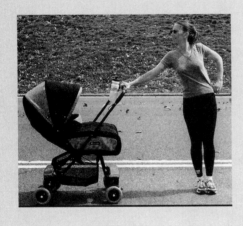 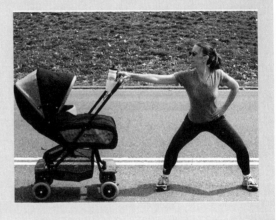

The Stroller Glide

This is a great butt-toning move.

1. Start with both hands on the stroller.

2. Step forward with your right leg, and push the stroller away from your body.

3. Now tighten your buns, and extend your left leg behind you (but don't lift it too high). Focus on lifting your leg, rather than swinging it back. Glide forward gracefully and avoid jerking the stroller. Be sure to keep your tummy tight, and don't arch your back.

4. When you've had enough of the Gliding Stroll, return to the Basic Stroll.

You should feel the sensation up the back of your legs into your buttocks. If you feel any tension in your lower back, it means that you're arching your back. Lower your leg, adjust your form, and try again. After a few minutes of this stroll, check your heart rate and compare it to your target heart rate on the chart (see page 95).

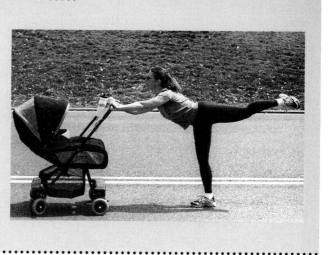

The Pull 'n' Roll

Here is a stroll that will come in handy whenever you have to back through a door with your stroller. It's also a favorite among the toddler set because they get to ride backward!

1. Keep both hands on the handlebar at all times.

2. Start by looking over your left shoulder, and stroll carefully backward, pulling the stroller along with you.

3. After a few seconds, turn your head to look over your right shoulder. Keep your chest open, and don't forget your Strollercize posture.

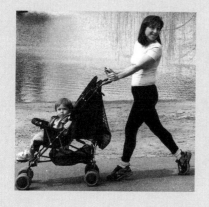

This stroll strengthens your quadriceps muscles, helps knee pain, and tones the tush. Pull the stroller with some force (but carefully—you're walking backward), and you'll get a great upper-body work-out as well. Don't do this stroll in a crowded area or on rough terrain. And never take your eyes off the road.

STROLLER STOPS AND STARTS

You've got the form, you're breaking a sweat. And just when you're feeling like nothing could stop you, you hit a red light. The following exercises are great for street corners, traffic lights, and any other time you need to stop for a few seconds. You can also incorporate these moves into an interval training program (see page 108). After four or five minutes of brisk strolling, do one or two minutes of any one of these moves, then start strolling again.

These moves will keep your heart rate soaring, while keeping your little bundle of joy entertained. Shoot for at least twenty-five repetitions of each exercise or thirty seconds, whichever comes first. Don't forget to lock the wheels of your stroller when you're parked, and keep the baby out of the sun. Some of these moves can get bouncy, so hold your breasts to protect them. I hope you've been doing your pelvic floor exercises (see Chapter 5). These are the moves that will remind you how weak or strong your pelvic floor muscles actually are.

Block the Baby

This is one of the most popular moves in Strollercize, and it comes in handy when you're trying to block your toddler from racing for that cookie jar (or worse). This exercise stretches the inner thighs and tones the abdominals.

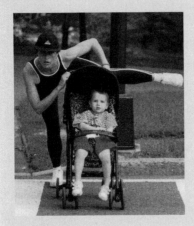

1. Keeping both hands on the handlebar, raise your left leg out to the side as high as it will go, and "block" the baby. Be sure to keep your lower back straight.

2. Bend forward at the knees, keeping your abdominals pulled in tight, and your knees directly over your ankles.

3. Switch sides.

Do at least 25 reps.

• • • • •

You'll really need to stretch your legs to get the benefits of this exercise.

Patty Cakes

Get ready to clap your hands and give the baby her first music lesson. You'll get a great stretch in your chest and shoulders. And the baby might even do a little clapping of her own.

1. Lock the stroller, and stand in front of the baby.

2. Lift your left leg to the front and bend your knee, as if you were looking at the sole of your shoe.

3. As you do this, clap your hands together under your leg.

4. Now lower your leg and stand up straight, clapping your hands behind your back.

5. Lift your right leg and repeat. Keep your chest lifted and your standing leg as stretched as possible.

Repeat 20 times or until you and baby are finished giggling.

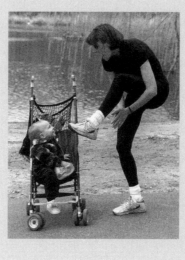

Hopscotch

Remember playing hopscotch as a child?

1. Lock the stroller.

2. Stand with your feet together and with your arms across your chest to protect your breasts.

3. Jump with your feet slightly apart, 6 to 8 inches.

4. Jump on only your right foot.

5. Jump on both feet again.

6. Jump on only your left foot.

7. Finally, jump again on both feet.

Repeat this sequence as rapidly as possible for 25 jumps or 30 seconds.

• • • • •

This exercise builds coordination and balance while keeping your heart rate up in your target zone.

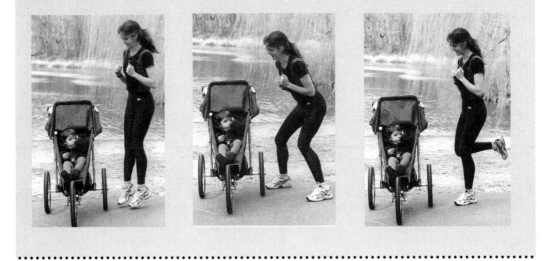

Rocking Horse

Look—Mommy is a pony! Feel free to whinny and neigh as you make like that nursery favorite.

1. Hold on to the stroller with your right hand. Be careful not to put a lot of weight on the handlebar.

2. Rock forward onto your left leg as you extend your right leg behind you, keeping both knees slightly bent.

3. Rock backward by shifting your weight back to your right foot and lifting your left leg. Both knees should be soft, your butt should be sticking out, and your abdominals should be tight. If you're doing this right, the baby will be able to tickle your toes when you rock forward.

4. Continue to rock forward and back for a while, then switch to the other side of the stroller and repeat. Your total time of "horsing around" should be 30 seconds for this stroller stop.

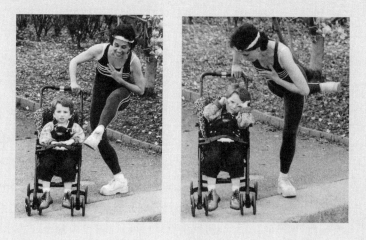

Ring Around the Stroller

This is a great way to play with the baby while freeing yourself from the stroller! It's simple. Just jog around the stroller. You baby will love watching you go. Do a few laps in one direction, then switch so you don't get dizzy. Grab the baby's rattle to keep your rhythm while you keep that heart rate soaring.

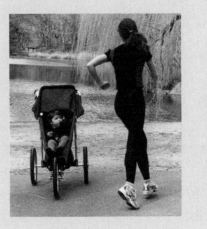

Tantrums

This is another Strollercize favorite. Let's say you've been listening to your toddler whine for hours on end. Now it's your turn to throw a tantrum. If you do this exercise frequently, you'll burn off some serious calories. And of course, the baby will love watching Mom go crazy.

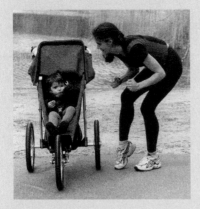

1. Begin to patter your feet on the ground.

2. Gradually increase the pace until your legs are moving very fast. Your pelvis should be tipped out, your chest up, and your tummy pulled in tight. As your feet move, your upper body will bend forward at the hips. Let your arms flay freely with the movement, or keep your arms over your breasts for protection. Once you're moving at full speed, keep it up for at least 30 seconds.

• • • • •

Good work, Mom! Next time the baby throws a tantrum you'll be ready to join in.

Progress Report

So you've been strolling for a few weeks, and you're wondering if you're making progress. To get to the "heart of the matter," a great measure of fitness is how fast your heart rate drops, or recovers, after a workout. Here's a simple test:

1. Stroll until you reach your target heart rate.

2. Stop strolling and march in place, slowly, for one minute. (Use your watch to time yourself.)

3. Now check your heart rate again, and see how much it's slowed down. A good result would be a steady rate of 16 beats or lower (based on a 10-second count).

· ·

RAISING THE INTENSITY

At first, you may feel so out of shape that even the warm-up knocks you out. But trust me, it will get easier. After a month or so, you'll probably be ready for a tougher workout. Here are some fun and easy ways to increase the intensity of your workout:

Pick Up the Pace. I probably don't need to tell you that the faster you stroll, the harder you'll work. That's why Strollercize recommends that you aim for a nice brisk pace (between 3.5 and 4.5 miles an hour). Most novice strollers can handle at least three miles per hour, and some speed-walking moms can cover as many as five miles in an hour. Use your heart rate as your guide. The idea is to start at the pace that is comfortable for you, and to go from there. When you feel ready to speed things up, figure out how long it takes you to complete your regular course. Then pick up the pace and try to beat your own record. Remember to increase your speed gradually, and always pace yourself.

I firmly believe that walking at a brisk pace is all that you need to do to build and maintain your aerobic fitness. There's really no need to break into a jog. In Strollercize we never run, because those ordinary four-wheeled strollers just can't take it. Plus, jogging can be very hard on your body, especially in those early months when everything's still weak and loose. If you're dead set on running during your Strollercize workout, do yourself a favor and invest in a jogging stroller (see page 42). And please take it easy.

Head for the Hills. Strolling up and down hills is another great way to add intensity to your workout. On the way up, you'll strengthen your hamstrings and challenge your heart. On the way down, you'll tone your quadriceps and calves. Great uphill moves include the Basic Stroll and the Rolling Stroll. And the Miniskirt is great for downhill. But never run downhill, as it's hard on your knees and can be dangerous for you and the baby.

Strollercize to a Faster Beat. If you have chosen to listen to music, try strolling to a faster beat. Just be sure to keep only one ear plugged into the music. You'll need your other ear to listen for the baby and traffic.

Try High-Low, or Interval, Training. Like your postpartum emotions, with high-low training you alternate between periods of working at a very high intensity and working at a lower intensity. In the gym, they call this interval training. It not only feels more intense, but some experts believe that it burns more calories than does maintaining a constant intensity. Plus, high-low training is a great way to beat the boredom factor.

During each interval, you should be working at about 80 percent of your maximum heart rate. The duration between intervals should be twice as long as the duration of the interval. (For example, a 45-second interval is matched with a 90-second recovery period.)

If timing yourself sounds too complicated, you can try out the landmark approach. Pick out a landmark (like a tree or a stop sign) a reasonable distance away, and then go forward full speed ahead. When you reach your landmark, slow down and catch your breath. Then pick a new landmark, and get moving again.

COOLING DOWN

Okay, you've given it your all, and you're ready to call it quits. But no matter how bushed you feel, don't stop moving suddenly. Slow down gradually. Remember, your heart and lungs are still working extra hard to get all that oxygenated blood to your muscles. Stopping suddenly can cause the blood to pool in your extremities, making you feel dizzy, nauseated, or even faint.

If you absolutely must stop strolling, march in place until your heart stops pounding and the sweat stops pouring. And don't even think about sitting down until your heart rate is at or below 50 percent of your maximum heart rate. Now is a great time to do a muscle-conditioning workout (see Chapter 8). But if you don't have the time, you should still finish off your aerobic workout with the stretches in Chapter 9.

8

Bootie Camp

This chapter presents the muscle-conditioning component of your Strollercize workout, Bootie Camp. The following moves will give you a total-body workout. You'll tone up the flab, while gaining the strength you need for daily activities. You'll also increase your muscle mass and raise your metabolism. You don't need weights or any other special equipment. You'll use the stroller for balance and your own body weight for resistance.

For the best results, you should do this Bootie Camp routine at least twice a week. Once you get the hang of it, you should be able to complete the entire workout in about twenty minutes. Unless otherwise specified, aim for ten to twenty repetitions of each exercise. Start at a level that's comfortable for you, and work up from there. Do as many repetitions of each move as it takes you to really feel your muscles working. You'll know it's time to stop when you can barely do another rep. After about three weeks, if you've been doing the program consistently, you should be able to complete twenty repetitions of each exercise. These moves are meant to be tough. So if you've done twenty reps (or more) and you still don't feel anything, you're not doing it right. Check your form and try again.

Remember that you should always warm up before you start your Bootie Camp routine. Do your Strollercize warm-up (see Chapter 6), or just run around with your toddler for five or ten minutes. The important thing is to warm up your body's core temperature before you move on to the more serious exercises.

Training Tips

The following tips will help you get the most out of your Strollercize muscle-conditioning workout.

- *Always warm up before your begin your routine, and cool down afterward. This helps prevent injuries.*
- *Exhale on the exertion (i.e., the hard part of the exercise), inhale naturally, and never hold your breath.*
- *Maintain good postural alignment. (Use the Strollercize Posture Checklist on page 57.)*
- *Working out has a discomfort factor. You will feel tired. The muscle will burn. You need to feel these sensations to get results. Of course, if you experience severe pain, then something is wrong. Stop immediately. Consult your doctor if the pain persists.*
- *Listen to your body. If something doesn't feel right, then stop. It's better to be safe than to risk a serious injury. If the pain persists, see your doctor.*
- *In general, you should do ten to twenty repetitions of each exercise. Start at ten and work up. But don't go crazy. You don't want to be so sore the next day that you can't take care of the baby!*

THE BOTTOM HALF

With all the focus on your growing belly during your pregnancy, you may not have noticed that the rest of your body was growing too. Now that the baby is born, it's harder to miss your newly enlarged legs, hips, and buttocks.

This workout will help you whip those lower body muscles back into shape. The exercises can be performed indoors or out. All you need is your stroller or a chair. For safety reasons, unless otherwise specified, make sure that the wheels of the stroller are locked while you perform these moves.

While the exercises are designed for use with a stroller, a sturdy chair will work in a pinch. Always do the moves in the order in which they are presented. You'll get a better workout and avoid injury.

Stroller Squats

This move will keep your lower body strong and your hips, thighs, and buttocks looking good. It also comes in handy when you have to squat down to pick up the baby, or to get up off the sofa. Before you begin, unlock the wheels of the stroller.

1. Stand behind the stroller, with both hands on the handlebar and your feet inside the wheels.

2. When you're ready, sit way back so your weight is on your heels, and your buns are level with your knees. If you're doing this right, you should be able to slide a piece of paper under the front of your shoes. The stroller may roll away from you so hold on tight.

3. Squeeze your pelvic floor muscles and your buns. Hold here for 10 counts.

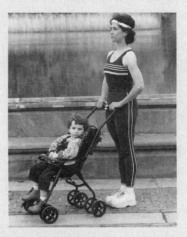

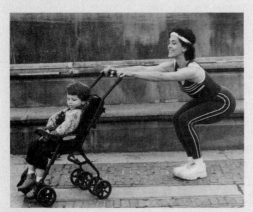

4. On your next exhale, press your heels into the ground as you raise yourself slowly back to your standing position.

5. Bring the stroller handlebar back toward your hipline using your arms, and stand tall with energy and tautness.

6. Repeat the movement.

Aim for at least 10 reps.

. . . . .

For best results, keep your buns tight and lifted through the entire exercise. Keep your shoulders down and relaxed, and your wrists straight. Your chin should be lifted, and your abs should be pulled in toward your spine for support.

Stroller Lunges

Lunging may be the least-loved exercise on the planet, but it is also one of the most effective. This move will tone your legs, buns, and hips. It will also give you the strength you need to pick up toys, scrub the floors, and push the stroller. Unlock the wheels of the stroller before you begin.

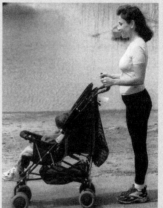

1. Start by placing both hands on the stroller handlebar. Find your Strollercize posture.

2. Now step forward with your left foot, and let the stroller roll out in front of you. As you step into the lunge, don't let your right knee touch the ground. You are in the correct position if your left knee is above your ankle, your shoulders are over your hips, and your right heel is over the ball of your right foot.

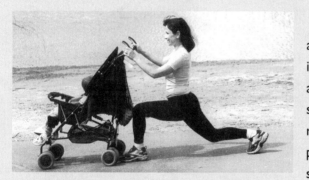

3. Try to tighten your buns, and drill the ball of the right foot into the ground behind you. As always, your wrists should be straight, your shoulders down and relaxed, and your chin up and proud. Be glad that you have the stroller to hold on to.

4. On your next exhale, tighten your pelvic floor muscles, and return to standing. Find your Strollercize posture.

5. Do as many repetitions as you can on your right leg. On the last rep, hold the lunge position for 10 counts.

6. Switch legs.

•••••

To intensify this move, take a bigger step forward, but do not sacrifice your posture. You may have to stagger out of this move, as your legs will probably feel like Jell-O—but isn't it better than having them look like Jell-O?

Stroller Roll-Outs

This move is a takeoff on the classic "dead lift" from the gym. It involves bending forward from your hips—something you'll probably do at least fifty times a day. Do it wrong, and you'll end up with lower back pain. Strollercize makes this complicated move safe and effective by using the stroller for support. This exercise will strengthen your back and is essential to getting through your daily "obstacle course" (see Chapter 10). Plus, this move will tone up that unwanted gunk on the backs of your legs. Before you begin, unlock the wheels of the stroller.

1. Stand with your hips square to the back of the stroller. Find your Strollercize posture.

2. Soften your knees slightly, and tilt your pelvis forward, just a tad.

3. Slowly push the stroller away from you as you bend forward from the hips. Don't move your feet. If you're doing this right, you will look like a table. Your back must be flat, and your wrists straight. Your eyes should be focused above the bar of the stroller, and your chest should be lifted. Keep your abdominals pulled in, but don't tuck your butt in. You will feel an incredible stretch in your back and hamstrings.

4. Now exhale as you gently lift your fingers off the stroller 1 inch, hold for 1 count, then lower. Do 10 to 20 reps.

5. When you've finished, keep your chest lifted and stand up into your Strollercize posture.

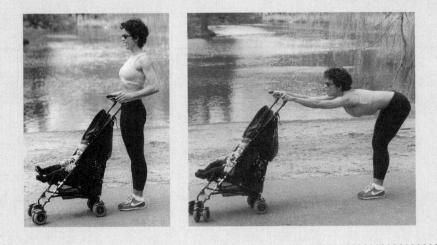

Step-Ups

After Tatiana was born, I was so desperate to get my lower body back that I found myself doing this move on the steps of the Plaza Hotel (about fifty times!). Sure, I may have looked a little silly, but this exercise is serious work for the butt, legs, and torso. It also helps to improve balance and coordination. FYI: This move is really intense, so please pace yourself.

To do this move, you'll need to find a sturdy park bench, chair, step, or bleacher. Look for a platform that's between 7 and 15 inches high, depending on your height: do not step up higher than a 90-degree angle at the knee. And make sure that the platform you choose is secure and not wobbly. Once you've found a place to step, position the stroller so that the baby can watch the show.

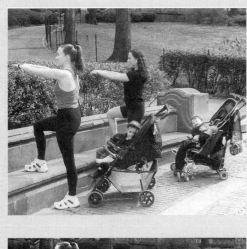

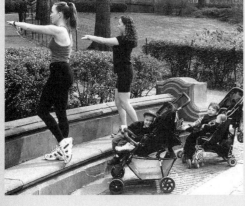

1. Start by placing your right foot up on the bench. Make sure your whole foot is on the bench.

2. Raise your arms out in front of you, and imagine that they are wrapped around a big tree. Lock your fingertips together.

3. Now try to hoist your body up without losing your form. Exhale as you rise to the top of the bench.

4. Once you're up, let your left foot dangle close to your right ankle.

5. Pretend your butt is a wet sponge, and give it a squeeze to get the water out. (But do not tuck your butt in.) Keep your abs pulled in tight against your spine.

6. Once you're up there, you may sway like a tree blowing in the wind. Use the strength of your torso muscles to keep your balance. Hold and balance for 5 counts.

7. Keep your right foot planted on the bench as you slowly lower your left foot to the ground. To protect your back, be sure to place your left foot as close to the bench as possible.

Do 10 to 20 reps on your right leg, then switch sides.

Saddle the Bag

I hate the term *saddlebags*. But I am all too familiar with the big bag of fat that loves to gather on my hips and thighs. Fortunately, Strollercize has a solution. This move will "saddle the bag."

1. Start with both hands on the stroller for balance.

2. Shift your weight to your right leg, and soften that knee slightly.

3. Raise your left leg to the side, slowly, until your foot is level with your knee.

4. Hold here for 10 counts.

5. Now slowly lift your foot even higher (aim for hip level), and then exhale as you lower your leg back to the height of your knee. Do 10 to 20 reps.

6. Now repeat the entire sequence on the same side.

When you have completed two sets, switch legs.

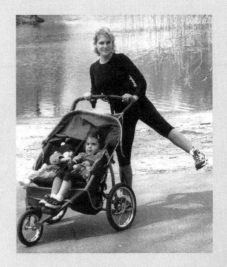

For best results, keep your shoulders square to the stroller, and try to stand tall as you lift your leg to the side. Keep a loose grip on the handlebar; this exercise is very hard, and I've seen moms hanging on to their strollers for dear life. For best results in working that saddlebag area, rotate your leg inward so that your foot points down to the ground. This will tone the area in no time. Big tip: The more relaxed the foot of your lifted leg, the more you'll target those saddlebags!

The T-Time

This move targets that glob of fat on the back of your buttocks and lower back. You'll also stretch your hamstrings, strengthen your lower back, and tighten your tummy. Before you start, unlock the wheels of the stroller so your arms will get involved too.

1. Stand behind the stroller in your Strollercize posture.

2. Slowly raise your left leg directly behind you until you can't lift it any more. You will feel a crimping sensation in your low back and waist. This is a normal feeling.

3. Once your leg is as high up as you can get it, lean forward and push the stroller away from you. Your shoulders should be square with the stroller.

4. Now slowly lower your left leg to the ground, and stand all the way back up as you pull the stroller back to your starting position. This movement should be slow and deliberate. Keep your left foot relaxed.

Do 10 to 20 reps. On the last rep, hold your leg in the air and pulse it up even higher for 20 counts. Repeat with your other leg.

• • • • •

Keep your back still during the entire exercise, and keep your buns tight.

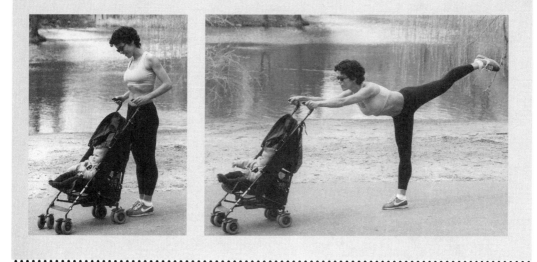

The Chunky Wunky

Are you afraid to let anyone catch a glimpse of you from behind? We understand. After having a baby, there is a spot on the back side of your waistline where the fat seems to settle. I call this area the "chunky wunky," because it's like an additional chunk of your body. This move will blast it away. Before you begin, lock the brakes on your stroller.

1. Stand facing the stroller in your Strollercize posture, with your hips touching the handlebar. Be sure to keep your hips glued to the bar for the whole exercise, to avoid twisting your spine or pelvis.

2. Put your left foot on the back of your right ankle. Harden your butt, and keep it perky. Gently turn your head to the left and look at your butt.

3. Now slowly lift your left leg about 6 inches away from your right ankle. Pulse the leg 10 times, then hold the leg steady for 10 counts.

Repeat this pulse-and-hold sequence 20 times, then switch sides. Be sure to keep your tush tight during the entire exercise. Work up to 50 reps.

• • • • •

You will really feel this in your outer butt, or the area that I call the "butt cuts" (that nice, defined line that cuts through the side of the glutes and looks great in skirts, pants, and leggings).

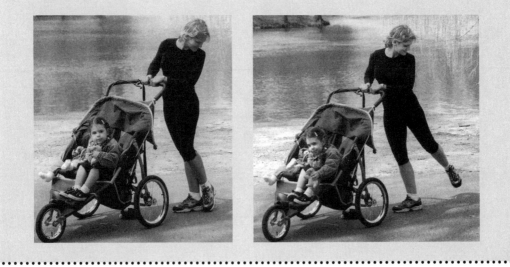

The Stroller Kickstand

Here's an exercise that will help improve your balance, strengthen your thighs, and prevent knee pain.

1. Stand along the left side of the stroller, and hold on to the handlebar with your right hand. Keep your wrist straight, your elbow up, and your shoulders down and relaxed.

2. Place your left hand on your hip with your elbow out to the side. Put all of your weight on the right foot, keeping your toes pointing forward.

3. Now extend your left leg out in front of you, and flex your ankle. Keep your left heel on the ground, as you straighten your left leg to really engage your thigh muscles. Check your posture: Your butt is tipped out, your spine is neutral, and your tummy is pulled in tight against your spine.

4. Now with the left toe pointing straight up, lift your left heel about 6 inches off the ground. Hold for 10 counts.

5. Slowly lower the heel to the ground, and then lift it right back up. Do 10 to 20 reps.

6. Take a quick rest and repeat on the same leg. And don't forget to switch sides.

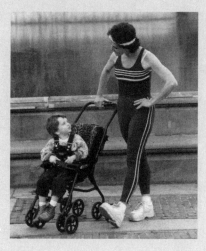
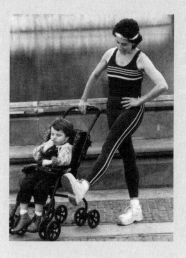

YOUR WAISTLINE

In this part of your Bootie Camp workout, you will use the stroller to melt inches off of your waistline and flatten your tummy. You will strengthen your abdominal and back muscles to help fight back pain.

Half of the exercises are done standing, and the other half are done on a bench. If you have time, unfold a blanket, camp out under a tree, and do the Waist Away routine from Chapter 5.

When you first do these exercises, you may feel some tightness in your lower back. This is normal—it usually takes about four sessions to loosen up the lower back. So stick with it!

Finding Your Waistline—Standing

As you may remember from Chapter 5, before you can reshape your waistline, you have to find it! Return to this basic move whenever you need a break.

I. The first step in Finding Your Waistline is to find your Strollercize posture. Get very close to your stroller so your hipbones touch the handlebar. This will help you isolate your abdominal muscles.

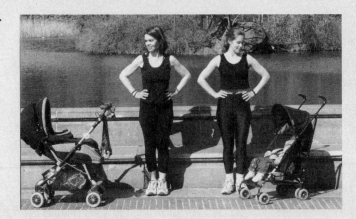

2. Now imagine that you're squeezing into your tightest pair of jeans. As you pull up that zipper, pull in your stomach using the transverse abdominal muscle. Find your waistline: Put your hands around your waist and see if you can touch your fingers around it.

3. Lift your chest up high, and try to get your hands deep inside your body. Close that diastasis (if you have one). Imagine that you are sewing up the seam of a corset.

4. Now release completely, and let your gut hang out. Repeat as needed.

Ding Dongs

Before you start, unlock the wheels of the stroller.

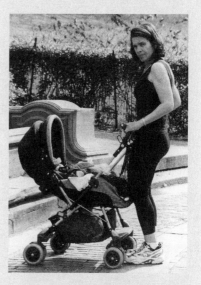

1. Rest your hipbones against the stroller, and place your fingers loosely on the handlebar.

2. Tuck your buttocks under your torso (this is the one time in Strollercize when you are allowed to tuck in your tail), and see if you can roll the stroller forward with your hips.

3. Now, if you pushed it forward, do it again. Keep a light touch on the stroller, and don't go crazy—you're not on the disco floor!

•••••

This movement will open up your lower back and isolate the abdominal muscles. Do 10 to 20 reps.

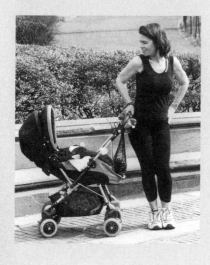

Variation: Turn sideways, and see if you can do your Ding Dongs that way. This move will incorporate the obliques and the side-of-the-waist area. Pretty soon you'll be able to wrap that belt around your waist again.

The Waister

This is a winner of a waistline exercise. And it's guaranteed to stroll away all that excess belly fat. Unlock the wheels of the stroller before you begin.

1. Stand sideways with your right hip next to the stroller and your right hand on the handlebar. Bend your knees slightly, and find your Strollercize posture.

2. Put your left hand on your left hip. Gently bend to the right, letting the stroller roll as far away from you as possible. You will feel an incredible stretch on the left side of your torso as you stretch and tone your obliques.

3. Now keep hold of the stroller as you lift back up. Take a peek at the baby. Exhale as you return to the starting position.

4. Do it again, and this time try to touch the top of your right arm to your right ear.

Do 10 to 20 reps, then switch sides.

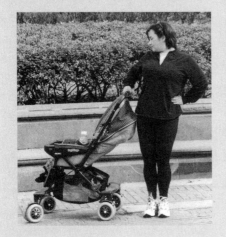 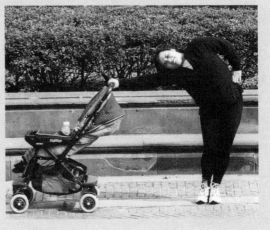

Check It Out

When you stroll, it's important to keep your eyes on the road. But that doesn't mean you can't check out the view from time to time.

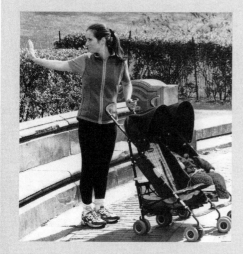

1. Stand in your Strollercize posture, with your hips touching the stroller. Put your left hand on the handlebar by your left hip. Bend your right arm to 90 degrees, and lift the elbow to shoulder height. This exercise works the obliques.

2. Now slowly twist around to the right, while keeping those hipbones glued to the stroller. Is there anything interesting behind you?

3. Exhale as you twist back to starting position.

4. Now try the other side—maybe there's something interesting over there.

Repeat 10 to 20 times.

• • • • •

The key to this exercise is to isolate the abdominals. Your chest may start to sink, so remember to keep it raised.

Crankies

This exercise is going to be tough, and it may make you feel cranky. But it's guaranteed to whip your waist into shape.

1. Face the stroller, and hold on with both hands. Find your Strollercize posture. Soften the knee of your right leg.

2. Bend your left leg, trying to touch your left foot to your butt.

3. Now lift the left leg (keeping it bent) to the side, trying to touch your outer thigh to your left elbow. For best results, don't lean away from the lifted leg, and con-

centrate on the contraction of muscles on your left side.

4. Now lower your leg about one inch, then bring it back up to your elbow. Repeat 10 to 20 times.

5. On the last repetition, hold your leg up for 10 counts.

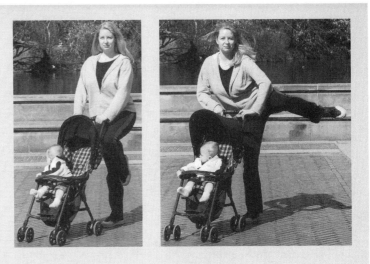

Do another set, and then get cranky on the right side.

Finding Your Waistline—Seated

First find a place to sit down. You may already be near a bench. Or if you're indoors, you can do this move while sitting on your sofa. Exercise is everywhere!

This is basically the same as Finding Your Waistline—Standing, except that you're going to feel even more flesh doubling up around your midsection.

1. Lift up your chest to stretch out that skin, and get those hands around your middle.

2. Try to get narrow in the waistline and regain your posture.

• • • • •

You should come back to this basic move in between each of the following exercises to give your back muscles a break.

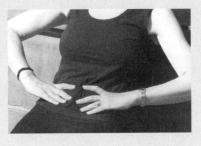

The Tummy Rumble

This move may be simple and sweet, but it's serious work for your tummy. Just be careful not to overdo it. Keep the stroller very close to you so you can give the baby a little jiggle as you work—and try not to worry if your tummy's jiggling too.

1. Sit on the very edge of the sofa or bench, with your legs extended and your knees slightly bent. Your feet should be gently touching the ground, directly in front of your knees.

2. Slowly sit back, rounding your back until the base of your shoulder blades touches the back of the bench. In fitness, this is called the "C curve." You need a strong C curve to protect your back and target the abs. You should feel your abs straining to sustain this position. If, however, you feel any strain in your back, you are probably not rounding your back enough. Stop, reposition, make sure you are sitting at the edge of the bench, and start again.

3. Now gently pitter-patter your toes on the ground. Keep your thighs relaxed, to really isolate those abdominal muscles. If you are doing this right, your tummy will rumble and shake. (If you have had a C-section, close your eyes and visualize the area where the incision was. Pull in on the scar, and see if you can activate that numbing sensation you experienced just after the surgery.) Count to 10.

4. Sit up, and Find Your Waistline.

Repeat the Tummy Rumble again. As you get stronger, you can increase your count to 20 but don't strain yourself.

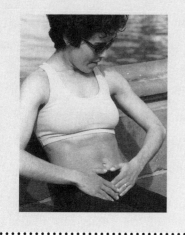
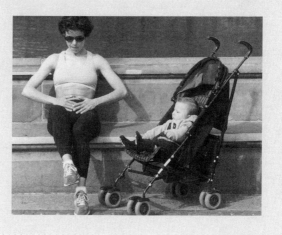

Pickups

You're feeding the baby and the bottle drops—you pick it up. Then the burping cloth falls off your shoulder—and you pick it up. A toy falls to the ground—you pick it up. The good news is that all of those pickups will strengthen your obliques and whittle your waist back into shape.

1. Sit on the edge of the bench with your stroller directly in front of you, your knees in front of your hips, and your ankles directly below your knees.

2. Put your right hand on the stroller, and bend directly to the left side, allowing your left arm to touch the edge of the bench as you reach to the ground. Imagine that you are picking up a fallen toy or baby bottle. You need to touch all five fingertips to the ground to make this move effective.

3. On your next exhale, lift yourself back to the starting position.

Do at least 10 reps on the left side, and then do the right side.

•••••

Pull in your tummy the entire time, and Find Your Waistline before moving on to the next exercise.

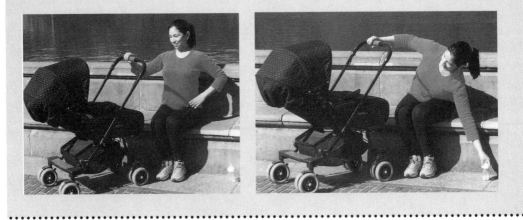

Switches

If you could switch a few things in life, what would they be? A new stroller? A new waist-line? Well, you may not be able to trade up. But this move will help you make the best of what you have.

1. Sit on the edge of the bench. Round your back, pull in your tummy, and make your C curve. Put your hands on the edge of the bench for support. Your shoulders may touch the back of the bench.

2. Bring your left knee into your chest, and stretch your right leg to the ground, pointing the toe.

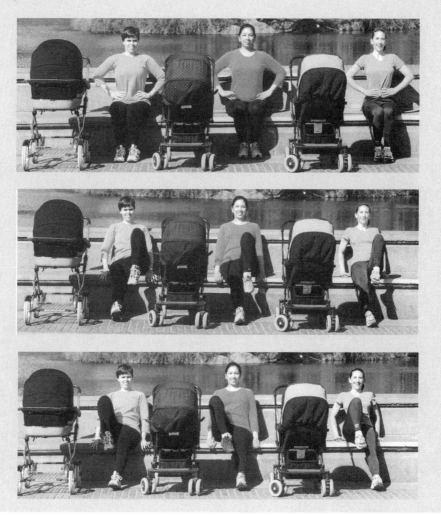

3. Hold this position for 10 counts and then switch your legs. Exhale on the switch.

Do 10 to 20 reps.

• • • • •

This may be the most effective exercise for the tummy. It will dig deep into your lower abdominals. But don't take my word for it. You'll feel the burn.

Kiss Knees

This exercise strengthens the core abdominal group, the rectus abdominus, and strengthens the back.

1. Sit on the edge of the bench, your legs in front of you, and round your back into a C curve, resting your back against the bench. Your shoulder blades should touch the back of the bench.

2. Touch your fingertips together, and bring your hands toward your mouth.

3. Gently bring your knees up toward your face, and try to give them a kiss. Hold this position for 10 counts.

4. Keep your toes pointed and your tummy tight as you lower your toes back down to the ground, close to the bench.

Shoot for 10 to 20 reps. Now sit up, and Find Your Waistline. When you are ready, do another set.

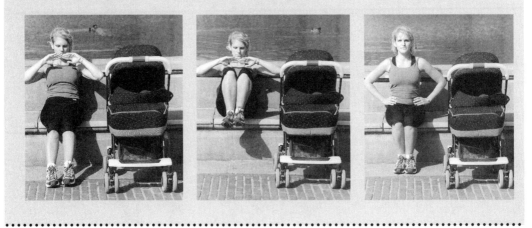

Kiss Knees Variation

This variation of Kiss Knees targets the sides of your waistline, which work the obliques. It's a bit more advanced, so you may need to work up to it.

1. Sit on your left hip, and twist your knees to the left.

2. Bring your right hand, palm out, to your mouth.

3. Lean back against the bench, and hold on with your left arm. Bring your knees toward your lips.

Do 10 to 20 reps, then switch sides.

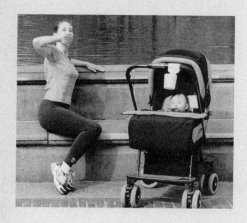 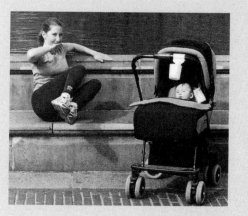

Tic Toc Waist

So you say you don't have time to exercise. Don't waste even a second thinking like that! Just sit your butt down, and Tic Toc that waist away. This move will tone your waist and help give you an hourglass figure.

1. Sit on the edge of the bench with your feet inside the wheels of the stroller. Put your left hand on the stroller and your right hand in the air.

2. Now bend to the left, reaching your right arm over your ear. Imagine that your arm is a dial on a huge clock, and see if you can reach all the way to nine o'clock. You

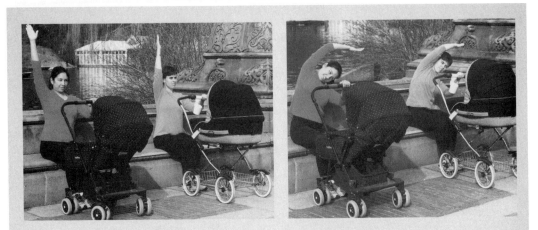

will feel a serious stretch on your right side and lots of little rolls of flesh creeping up to your bra on the left. Good. Keep bending.

3. Repeat on the other side, and try to find three o'clock.

Do 10 to 20 reps.

The Goddess Twist

1. Sit on the edge of the bench and Find Your Waistline. Cross your arms in front of you to form an X, resting your opposite hand on the opposite knee, your left arm on top.

2. Now take your left hand and reach upward as you twist your torso to the right. Take your time and luxuriate in the stretch.

3. Switch sides.

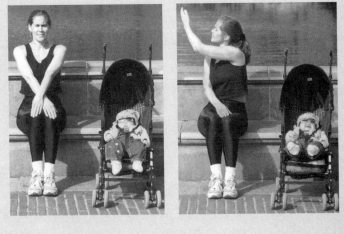

Do 10 to 20 reps.

MOM'S LOVING ARMS

Get off that bench and give your buns a break. It's time to tone the arms. Your daily life (pushing the stroller, lifting the baby, carrying the diaper bag) is already a serious upper-body workout. Here are some exercises to tone those muscles and train your upper body for the real workout that is your life. In most of the arm work, make sure the baby is watching you and the stroller wheels are braked.

The Curb

If you live in a big city, as I do, you'll run into plenty of curbs. And even if those pesky little steps aren't part of your daily life, you'll still appreciate the effects of this move on your triceps muscles. Before you begin, double-check to be sure that your baby is strapped securely into the stroller. This exercise can be done standing in line at the bank or shopping mall.

1. Stand facing the stroller, holding the handlebar with both hands. Bend your knees slightly, lean forward just a bit, and look at the baby.

2. Now imagine that you are approaching a very high curb. On your next exhale, gently push down on the handlebar and straighten your arms. The stroller will tilt back slightly. Keep your shoulders relaxed and down.

3. Return to the starting position by gently lowering the baby in the stroller so that the wheels land softly. Repeat.

Do 10 to 20 repetitions.

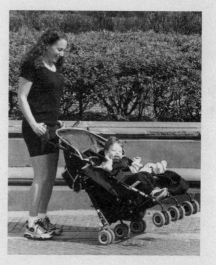

• • • • •

If you're lucky, the gentle, rocking motion will lull your baby to sleep.

Push-Ups

There is no two ways about it: The Push-Up is the best upper-body exercise on Planet Fit. Yes, it is hard, but please do not skip this exercise! You'll work your chest, arms, shoulders, and even your abs. Push-Ups can be done anywhere—off of a bench, a mailbox, a bleacher, a car, a couch. Just be sure the base you select is sturdy and secure. If you're really brave (and strong), hit the deck and do your Push-Ups on the ground. Before you start, make sure baby is facing you, as this is another very entertaining exercise.

1. Stand facing the bench. Place your hands on the back of the bench about 18 inches apart, or slightly wider than your shoulders. (To protect your wrists, you can form a triangle with the thumb and forefinger of each hand.)

2. Take a deep breath as you bend your arms, and lower your chest toward the bench. If you're in the correct position, your nipples should touch the bench.

3. Hold for a few counts, if you can.

4. Exhale as you straighten your arms and return to the starting position.

Work up to 20 to 40 Push-Ups.

.....

I am not kidding about the number of repetitions. At first you should do the move slowly. As you get stronger, you may want to alternate a set of slow Push-Ups with a quicker set. Working at a faster pace recruits additional muscles and can add to the benefits of this move.

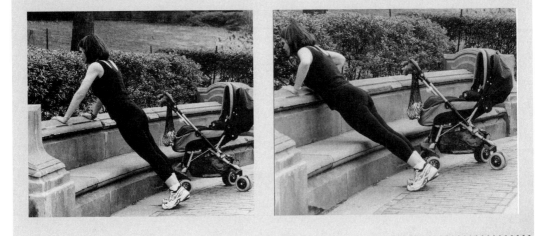

Stroller Dips

This exercise targets that stubborn flab on the backs of your upper arms. Although it's another great park bench move, you can also take it indoors to a sturdy chair or coffee table. Be sure to keep the stroller nearby so that the baby can watch the action.

1. Sit on the edge of the bench. Extend your legs straight out in front of you, with your feet in front of you.

2. Place the pads of your hands on the bench, at the sides of your hips, with your knuckles pointing toward your toes.

3. Now lift your body off of the bench and slide your buns forward, just past the edge of the bench. Your knees will bend.

4. Hold here for 10 counts.

5. Slowly lower your body toward the ground, until your arms make a 90-degree angle at the elbow joint. Keep your chin lifted, your shoulders down, and your chest up. Your buns should not be tucked, and there should be very little weight on your heels. Most of your body weight should be on your arms.

6. Once you reach the 90-degree point, push down into the bench with your hands and stretch your arms as you come out of your dip. Think of chocolate fondue and keep dipping!

·····

You should work up to two sets of 10 to 20 repetitions. Your arms will shake if you are doing this right—just think of it as "shaking" off all that unwanted flesh behind your arms.

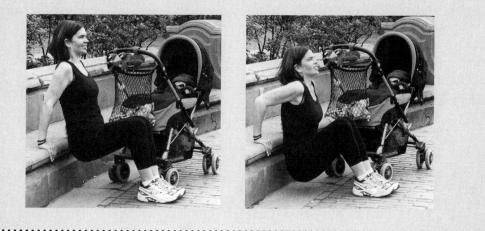

The One-Arm Push

This is a tough one, so you can skip it if you like. But as a mother of three who's used to doing everything with one hand, I've found that this exercise has made my day much, much easier. It's also done wonderful things to the shape of my arms.

You can do these pushes against a playground wall, high fence, or even a drainboard. When you get stronger, you can do it on the bench.

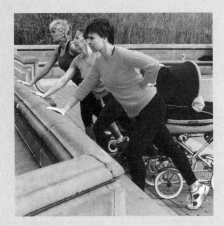

1. Place your right hand directly in front of the middle of your chest line, and point your right elbow out to the side. Put your left hand behind your back. Spread your feet wide so you have a solid base, and step your left leg forward for added support.

2. Bend the elbow of your right arm slowly, and see if you can get your left shoulder to touch the bench.

3. Exhale as you push away from the bench, and straighten your arm fully.

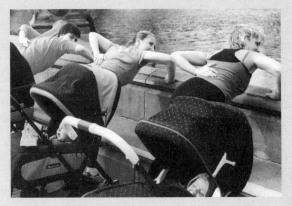

Start with just a few reps, and work up from there. And don't forget to switch arms.

Seated Rolls

Back to the bench, for another great upper-body move. In the gym, they call this exercise Seated Rows. But in Strollercize we call it Seated Rolls. It targets the shoulders and upper back.

1. Sit on the bench facing the stroller, with its wheels unlocked. Put your left foot on the footrest of the stroller, and both hands on the handlebar.

2. Push the stroller away so your arms extend directly out in front of your shoulders. Your left leg will be stretched too.

3. Now apply some resistance with your foot, as if you were pushing on a bike pedal, and try to bring the stroller handlebar back to your chest. Keep your elbows up at shoulder level, your chest lifted, and your chin up. Your back should be straight—try not to slouch.

. . . . .

This exercise requires a very strong torso, so be sure you've mastered your abdominal routine (see Chapter 5) before attempting this exercise. Do 10 reps and enjoy the feeling in your arms and back.

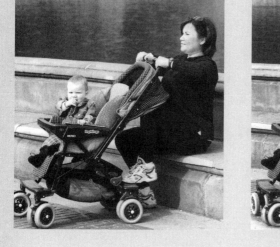 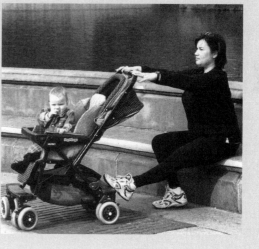

The Bosom Lift

You don't need a push-up bra to lift that sagging chest, but you do need this exercise. This move will perk up your bosom while strengthening your arms, shoulders, and back. Unlock the wheels of the stroller before you begin.

1. Sit on the edge of the bench with your legs apart and the stroller in front of you. Push the stroller out a bit so you can lean forward, and place your hands on the outside of the stroller. Keep your head down and check out your cleavage.

2. Now gently squeeze the frame of the stroller. You don't need to squeeze very hard to feel the contraction in your chest.

3. As you are squeezing, roll the stroller away from your body, then bring it back. Keep your tummy pulled in tight.

Do 10 to 20 reps. On the last rep hold the squeeze for 10 counts. Work up to 2 sets.

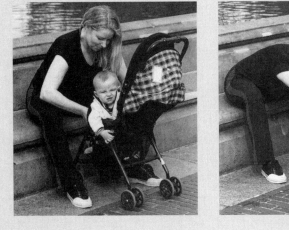 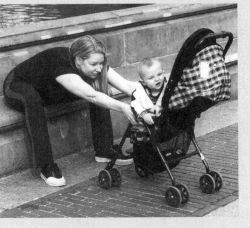

The Stroller Lift

You probably do this move a hundred times a day—like when you're lifting the wheels of a stroller to make a turn, or trying to fit between the tables of a cozy restaurant. It's also a great upper-body strengthener.

1. Sit on the edge of the bench, facing the stroller with your feet between the wheels.

2. Find Your Waistline.

3. Put both hands on the stroller, and raise your elbows out to the side, in line with your shoulders. Keep your chin lifted.

4. On your next exhale, slowly lift the stroller wheels a few inches off the ground using your shoulder muscles.

5. Lower the stroller wheels back down, gently.

Do 10 to 20 reps.

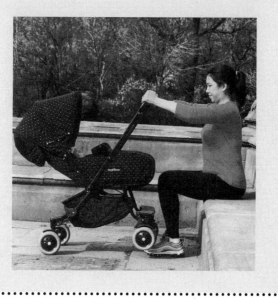

Playing the Pram

By now your arms should be feeling tired and heavy. And you may be thinking that you've had enough. Wrong! We're going in for the "cuts." This move will not only give you beautifully toned arms, it will help strengthen the wrists for pram pushing. You can do it standing or sitting.

   1. Raise your arms out to your sides, about shoulder height, and move your fingers in the air as if you were playing a piano. Move your fingers as fast as you can, and imagine that they are moving up and down the scale.

   2. Do this for at least a minute. Your shoulders will burn like crazy, your forearms will sizzle, and your fingers will start to feel numb. Try to keep those fingers moving for as long as you can stand it.

   3. Then go immediately to Wings, without putting your arms down.

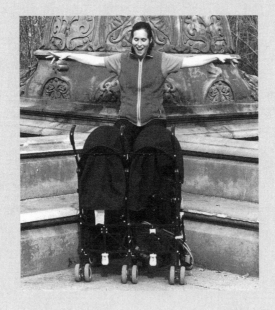

Wings

There are moments when every new mom wishes she had wings to carry her away. Although this move won't help you to fly, it will keep the flesh on your upper arms from flapping in the wind. You can either sit or stand for this exercise. But, either way, be sure to keep your Strollercize posture.

1. With your arms extended out to the side, relax your hands as if they were feathers. Tip your elbows up, making sure that they are in line with your shoulders.

2. Now slowly raise your arms up about two inches, then lower them back down to their starting position. Keep your back open and wide and your abdominals pulled in. Your chin should be lifted and your jaw loose. Keep your shoulders relaxed and away from your ears.

3. Continue lifting and lowering your arms for at least one minute. See the flab on your arms fly, fly away.

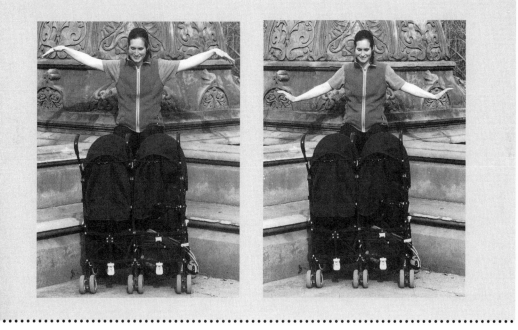

So there you have it—twenty-four of the best exercises a mom can do to get a total body workout. Yes, this routine is tough. But your life is tougher, and you need to train for it.

I know you're tired. But never too tired to stretch before you stroll home. Take a few minutes to stretch out your muscles so you won't be too sore tomorrow. Chapter 9 will help you loosen up and chill out.

9

Chilling Out

*L*ife is rarely predictable. And life with a baby is *never* predictable. Flexibility is essential to your new life, in both mind and body. The following moves will help you limber your body and open your mind. This is your time to relax, stretch your muscles, and feel good about yourself and what you've accomplished.

Stretching is an important part of your Strollercize program. You should take the time to stretch your muscles after each and every workout. I know you're busy, but skipping out on stretching is a dangerous way to save time. Not only will you be sore the next day, but you'll be setting yourself up for a serious injury. Stretching helps to elongate the muscles, which gives you a nice, toned appearance. Besides, stretching is relaxing, and you deserve to relax.

You should take each of the following stretches to the point of gentle tension. You will feel a gentle pulling sensation in the muscles. Try to hold each stretch for at least twenty or thirty seconds. (As you become more flexible, you may feel like holding some of the stretches for up to a minute.) Hold steady, and exhale into the tension. Don't bounce, as this can tear your muscle fibers.

In addition to your stroller, you will need a park bench, a sturdy chair, or some porch stairs. And be sure to lock the wheels of the stroller before you begin.

The Big-Breasted Breath

This deep-breathing move is a great way to relax your body and seal in the benefits of your workout. Perform this technique whenever you start to feel that your life is too much to handle. This move will help you to cleanse your mind and put everything back into perspective.

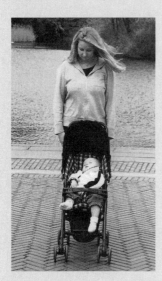

1. Start in a comfortable standing position in front of the stroller so the baby can see you, with your feet under your hips. Inhale slowly, as you let your arms float up to your sides until they are about chest level. Breathe into your lungs, not your stomach. Feel your torso filling up with air as your chest expands and your breasts grow bigger (as if that were possible).

2. When you are ready to exhale, let out a big "end of the day" sigh. Try to release as much air as you can (at least twice as much as you inhaled), and feel the tension and stress releasing from your body. Make as much noise as you need to. Don't hold anything back.

3. When you're finished, you should feel alert, relaxed, and ready to take on the world. Repeat as needed.

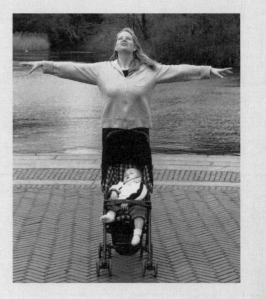

The Cereal Box Reach

This move comes in handy when you're trying to reach that box of rice cereal at the back of the cupboard. It's also a great stretch for your torso and arms.

1. Stand next to your stroller, with your left hand on the handlebar and your feet a hip width apart.

2. Raise your right arm, soften your knees, and reach for that cereal box. Lift up your chest and lean back, slightly. You should feel the stretch in your stomach and armpits. Reach for 20 seconds.

3. Switch sides.

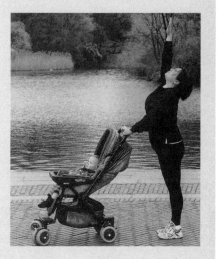

Baby Talk

What was that, Baby? Although he's probably not talking yet, this move will help you to hear all of those precious gurgles and grunts. Plus, it's a great stretch for your neck.

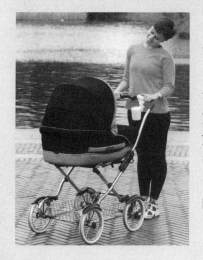

1. Stand behind the stroller, with both hands on the handlebar.

2. Now slowly tip your head to the left as if to touch your ear to your left shoulder. As you move your head, be sure to keep your shoulders down and your spine straight. You will feel a stretch along the right side of your neck.

3. Hold this position for a few seconds while you listen to your baby.

4. Switch sides.

Which Hand?

This move stretches your upper back and shoulders, and it is the perfect remedy for that sagging chest. It's also a great stretch for recovering your posture after breast-feeding. You should feel the stretch in your shoulders and back, along with a gentle contraction in your middle back.

1. Stand with your back to the stroller and your hands on the handlebar behind you.

2. Bend forward from your hips at about a 20-degree angle. Keep your chest slightly lifted, and squeeze your shoulder blades together. (For an added stretch, turn to the left or right and sneak a peek at baby.) Your knees should be slightly bent and your hips neutral.

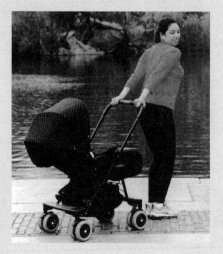

Hide-and-Go-Peek

This is not only a fun game to play with the baby but a serious total-body stretch.

1. Stand behind the stroller, with both hands on the handlebar. Your feet should be as wide apart as possible (at least wider than the wheels of the stroller), with the toes pointing forward.

2. Now stick your tush out behind you, as you bend your knees and lower your buttocks toward the ground. Try to get your rear end as close to the ground as possible without lifting your heels.

3. Contract your pelvic floor muscles. If you're doing this right, you'll be almost completely hidden behind the stroller. You should feel a serious stretch in your arms, shoulders, legs, and hips.

4. Take a few moments to enjoy the sensation, and then slowly straighten your knees and return to standing.

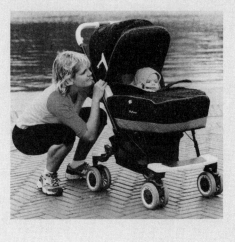

Swan Lake

This move will help you to feel as strong as a dancer and as graceful as a swan. You'll also feel a wonderful stretch in your waist, hips, and hamstrings. For this move, you'll need to find a park bench or a sturdy couch.

1. Stand facing the bench, holding the stroller with your right hand for balance.

2. Put your left heel up on the back of the bench, with your toes facing the sky. Your right leg should be slightly soft, and your toes should point toward the bench. Your hips must be even and not tilted to either side.

3. Now keep your chest lifted as you bend forward, reaching your left hand toward your left shin. To increase the stretch, see if you can walk your fingers down your leg to your toes.

4. Repeat on the right leg.

· · · · ·

Move the stroller as necessary.

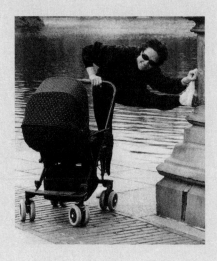

Leg Up!

1. Stand facing the stroller (a bench, high table, railing, or a fence will also work), holding the handlebar.

2. Put your left foot up on the handlebar.

3. Keep your chest lifted as you bend your left leg and lean into the stretch.

4. Switch legs.

•••••

If you do this exercise with the stroller, brace the stroller against a wall or other stationary object for safety.

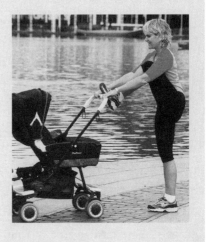

Toes-to-Nose

Your baby probably does this move all the time to get a taste of her toes. While you may not be as limber as a five-month-old, you will still reap the benefits of this wonderful stretch.

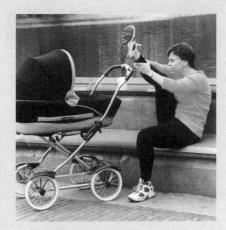

1. Sit on the bench and grasp your right ankle with both hands.

2. Slowly raise your foot up to your mouth and nose—or as close as you can. If you are superflexible, you may even be able to bring your leg over your neck. If necessary, let your upper body round forward, slightly, to bring your face closer to your foot. But keep your neck and shoulders relaxed. You should feel this stretch in your right hip.

3. Repeat on the left side.

•••••

Any questions? Watch the baby, she's a pro.

The Relaxed Roll-Out

This stretch is a simple variation of the Seated Rolls, from the Bootie Camp routine. After all that hard work, you'll love what this does for your upper body. Unlock the wheels of the stroller before you begin.

1. Sit on the edge of a park bench or sturdy chair, with the stroller a few inches in front of you. Your legs should be wide apart, and your feet should be outside the wheels of the stroller.

2. Hold on to the handlebar with both hands, keeping your elbows level with your shoulders and your chest lifted.

3. Roll the stroller forward as you bend forward from your waist. Relax your upper body, and let your head drop down between your knees. Don't get bummed out if you happen to catch a glimpse of your thighs on the way down. (Trust me, they look much bigger from this angle.) Just relax, and enjoy the stretch in your upper body and back.

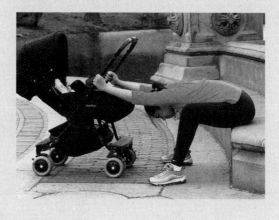

The Hangover

Despite the name, this move has nothing to do with that horrible morning-after feeling. In fact, this stretch will leave you feeling so mellow and content, you may even forget you've been up all night.

1. Start by sitting nice and tall.

2. Take a deep Big-Breasted Breath (see page 142).

3. On the exhale, relax your entire body, collapse forward slowly, and lower your head down between your knees. Let your arms hang down to the ground. (If it's more comfortable, rest your hands on your ankles.)

4. Hold this position, and enjoy the sensation.

5. When you are ready to rise, roll up as slowly as possible, straightening only one vertebra at a time. Be aware of any areas of tension, and let them release as you roll up. Your head and neck should come up last.

•••••

This final move will stretch and relax your whole body, as it seals in the benefits of your Strollercize workout. Take your time, and try to savor the moment. Even though your toddler is getting away! Breathe, mom, you deserve to relax.

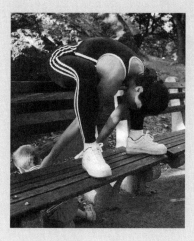

III

A Day in Your Life
· ·

Congratulations! You've made it through your Strollercize workout. But you're not finished yet. You still have to get through the rest of your day. Chapter 10 shows you how to navigate your daily obstacle course. From folding the stroller to lifting the baby, you'll learn how to get the most out of your everyday activities. In Chapter 11, I'll address moms' most common excuses for not exercising, and give you some tips for making Strollercize a permanent part of your new life.

..............10...............
Mom's Daily Obstacle Course

$\mathcal{M}$otherhood is hard physical work. From lifting the baby to pushing the stroller, you'll get plenty of exercise each and every day just going about the business of being a mom. The good news is that you'll be getting a workout without even trying. The bad news is that, if you're not careful, all of this extra work will take a serious toll on your body. In this chapter, I'll take you through a day in the life of a new mother and help you to navigate the obstacle course that is your new life.

THE STROLLER

All three of my children were born in the same New York City apartment: a sixth-floor walk-up. Yes, that meant I had to climb six flights of stairs day in and day out—through three pregnancies, with three newborn babies, and of course, with the stroller. But getting out of my building was only the beginning. New York City, like most of the world, is hardly stroller friendly. Once I was liberated from my home, I still had to worry about squeezing through narrow doorways, navigating through crowded department stores, bumping over curbs, and folding the stroller to jump on the bus. I had unwittingly entered the ranks of mothers who were disabled by their strollers.

By the time my third child, Romeu, was born, I was starting to get the hang of my new life. Here's what I've learned.

Doorways

For a mom with a stroller, a doorway is always a struggle. As with many mothers, your first attempt to push open a door with your stroller may have looked like a contortionist act in the circus. First, you pushed your stroller toward the door, hoping that it would magically open with a gentle tap from the stroller. Dream on. Next, you reached your arm over the stroller (which was still between you and the door), trying desperately to reach and then turn the knob. If your arms are very long and you actually managed to reach the door, you then had to push it open and steam-roll your stroller through the door before it swung shut again. I hope you and the stroller made it through in one piece!

Besides the low success rate of the aforementioned method, doing it repeatedly could lead to upper and lower back strain, twisted shoulder joints, and more than your share of frustration. Fortunately there is an easier way.

The Doorway: Pushing

The trick to pushing your way through a doorway is to avoid putting the stroller between yourself and the doorway. Here's how:

1. Turn yourself and your stroller around and move backward, pulling the stroller with you, toward the doorway.

2. Turn the doorknob, and use your whole body to push open the door.

3. Carefully step backward through the doorway, pulling your stroller along with you. With a spring door, you can use your body as a doorstop as you push the stroller through the door. Once the stroller has cleared the doorway, you can turn it around and go on your merry way.

The Doorway: Pulling

Now it's time to move on to an even bigger challenge—pulling the door open. This move really works your triceps and delts, so you'd better be training those muscles!

1. Back yourself and the stroller into the doorway. When you've made contact with the door, turn away from the stroller and open the door with your stronger arm.

2. With your free hand, pull the stroller halfway through the doorway, using your body to keep the door open. You should be between the door and the stroller; don't put the stroller in the middle.

3. Once the stroller has cleared the door opening, let the door close, turn the stroller around with both hands, and you're in!

Curbs

During your years of living without a stroller, you probably never noticed just how many curbs you encounter in the course of your day. Now, as a mom with a stroller, you can no longer ignore these annoying little bumps. Getting over a curb with a stroller is no easy feat. The most important thing to do when you encounter a curb is to take it slow. You do not want the baby to get knocked around in the stroller. And of course, you have to see that curb coming before you bump into it!

Going Up

1. As you approach a curb from the street, push down on the stroller handlebar to tilt the stroller backward and lift the front wheels. For extra leverage, place your foot on the footrest (if your stroller has one), and press down. Keep your wrists straight and your shoulders away from your ears.

2. Once the front wheels are up on the curb, lift the back wheels onto the curb, using your shoulders. (See Lifting Your Stroller on page 158.)

This move calls upon your triceps, biceps, and shoulders. The next time you hit that curb, you'll be thankful you did all of those Stroller Dips, Wings, Pull-Ups, and Push-Ups (see Chapter 8).

Going Down

Despite what you might think, strolling down off a curb is just as treacherous as strolling up. Many moms just plow down the curb, letting the front wheels of the stroller tip downward, as if they were emptying a wheelbarrow into the street. (I hope their babies are strapped in tight.) A better approach:

Use your triceps muscles to tip the front wheels up, as the back wheels gently roll down the curb. That way the stroller stays level, and you avoid jarring the baby.

Folding the Stroller

So you want to jump into the car, take a bus, or enter that cozy restaurant where there are "no strollers allowed." Well, Mom, it looks like you're going to have to fold up that stroller. With the wrong kind of stroller, this daily chore can be more than just a hassle—it can be your worst nightmare. First, consider that to fold most of the strollers on the market, you need to use two hands. That means that you have to find a safe place to put the baby (and all the stuff that was loaded into your stroller) while you fold it. Unless you have a friend to hold the baby or a car seat to put her in, you're out of luck. Second, most of the two-handed models on the market are ridiculously difficult to use. Some models are intellectually challenging, while others require that you have superhuman strength or perform ridiculous physical contortions.

If you've managed to purchase one of the few strollers on the market that can be closed with only one hand, congratulations! You have just saved yourself a lot of pain and aggravation. You may skip to the next section of this chapter, as the following information does not concern you. If you are like most moms, however, you may have to give up and ask a stranger to hold the baby, while you wrestle with the stroller. I suggest you try a "dry run" of these moves at home so that you can swing into action in public with no problem.

Folding the Stroller

With proper form, your legs, buttocks, and lower back muscles will do most of the work, lessening your chances of straining your shoulder and arms. The following steps should make things easier:

1. Find a safe place for the baby, away from the stroller, if possible. If you must hold the baby, carry her in your weaker arm. Be sure that those tiny hands and feet are out of the way. You don't want them to get caught in the stroller.

2. Stand a comfortable distance from the stroller, and bend at your hips until you are able to reach and activate the mechanism(s) for folding the stroller. As you bend forward, remember to keep your tummy tight, your knees soft, and your back flat. Your buttocks should be sticking out behind you, not tucked under your body. For some strollers, you can activate the mechanism with your feet, in which case you just need to lift your leg and flex those shin muscles.

3. Lunge down alongside the stroller so that you can fold it. As you lunge, be sure that your front knee is directly above your ankle, and your belly button is pressed tightly against your spine.

4. Gather the stroller into your hands. Keeping your knees bent, slowly bring your legs together and lift the stroller. Be careful not to tuck your butt under your torso or to round your back.

Lifting Your Stroller

I know what you're thinking: "Lift the stroller? Are you crazy?" Yes, your stroller is heavy, and no, I do not recommend performing this move on a daily basis. But there will be times when you'll have to lift that stroller (e.g., to carry it down stairs or over a big curb). Practice this move at home first, so you won't feel as embarrassed if you collapse under the weight of that four-wheeled monster in public.

Lifting Your Stroller

This move is based on two exercises from the Strollercize Bootie Camp routine (see Chapter 8): Stroller Lunges (see page 113) and Stroller Roll-Outs (see page 114). Learning to lift the stroller in this fashion enables a mom to see the ground in front of her. It also requires a lot of arm strength, so I hope you've been doing those Push-Ups. Be sure to take it easy, and have your husband or a friend spot you for your first couple of trys.

1. Turn the stroller so that the baby is facing you, and move alongside the stroller. Pick the side of the stroller that you feel the strongest to lift—usually the left side of the stroller.

2. Lunge down along the right side of the stroller, but try to avoid going into a kneeling position—it will take more strength to rise up. Now, gently lean forward, keeping your back flat, chin up, and tummy tight. Grab hold of the stroller with your left hand

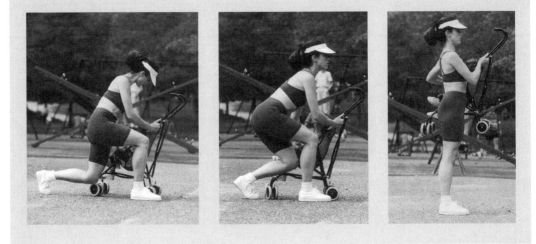

at the bottom metal side bar and your right hand on the top of the other side, directly diagonal to your left hand. (By the way, you can do this with the opposite approach if your other side is stronger.)

3. Keep your chin lifted and your biceps flexed as you lift the stroller up and rest it against your hip. Keep the stroller close to your body to help take the load off your back.

4. Stand up straight, and feel grounded. You are now holding about 50 pounds of stroller and baby (and that's if you took my advice and packed light). If anyone sees you do this move, they'll surely stop and applaud!

. . . .

Stairs

Just for fun, I spent an afternoon outside of New York's busiest toy store to get a firsthand look at moms with their strollers. I was especially intrigued by the three stairs leading up to the store's main entrance. I watched mother after mother try to carry their strollers and babies up and down the stairs. A few of the mothers, who were too weak to lift their strollers, resorted to dragging their strollers up the steps backward (giving their babies a terribly bumpy ride). The more patient mothers simply stood at the base of the stairs and waited quietly for someone to offer their assistance. Sometimes it took as many as four people to carry a single stroller up the stairs. And most of these mothers waited for a very long time for even one person to stop and help them.

The fact is that there is neither a safe nor an easy method of getting a stroller up or down stairs. You always risk tripping on the stairs and sending your baby down with the stroller. Moreover, getting a stroller over stairs is serious physical work. Unless you are built like Wonder Woman, you will inevitably strain your shoulders, arms, or back.

My best advice is: Whenever possible, stay away from places with stairs. If you can't avoid them, your safest bet is to fold the stroller and carry the baby in your arms. But there may be times when you absolutely must get the stroller up or down a flight of stairs. The following tips should make it a little less risky for you and the baby.

How Not to Do Stairs. The most common (and the worst) way to get a stroller over stairs goes something like this: You walk backward up the staircase as you pull the stroller in front of your body. Yikes! This method is an accident waiting to happen. First, since you can't see either your feet or the stairs, you are almost certainly going to trip. And if you do fall, you are standing behind the stroller, which leaves your baby completely unprotected.

How to Do Stairs

A safe way to get a stroller over stairs is as follows:

1. Turn the stroller so that your baby is facing you. This way if you trip, your body will act as a barrier between the baby and the floor.

2. Lunge down alongside the stroller (see Lifting Your Stroller on page 158). Your back should be straight, your tummy should be tight, and your buttocks should extend out behind your body.

3. Stretch your arms across the stroller (to act as an extra "seat belt"), and hold on to two sturdy, preferably metal, opposite parts of the stroller.

4. Lift the stroller, and rest it on your hip. With the stroller in this position, you'll get a clear view of the steps and will avoid overstressing your shoulders and back. As you move, you and the baby should practically be cheek-to-cheek.

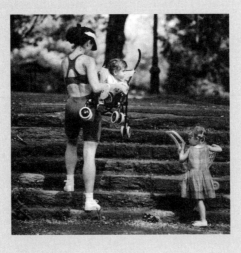

Elevators

Living up six flights of stairs, as I do, I've often wished for an elevator to make my life easier. And clearly for the average mom, carrying a stroller up even a single flight of stairs is not a practical option. But before you let out that big sigh of relief at the sight of an elevator, you should know that elevators are only slightly easier to navigate than the stairs.

How to Do Elevators

An elevator is a real sardine tin for a mom with a stroller. The following guidelines should help:

1. Always back into the elevator. Be sure to get all the way in so that you clear the doors. Elevator doors are equipped with sensors to stop them from closing on your stroller, but I've seen doors close on strollers anyway!

2. If possible, try to be the last one in the elevator, and plant yourself in front by the door. The people behind you can always squeeze around the stroller to get out. But get stuck in the back, and you'll have to steam-roll your way out of that crowded elevator.

3. Be brave! On a busy Saturday at Bloomingdale's, I watched mom after mom wait for an empty elevator, rather than take one that already had people in it. (In fact, I think a few of those moms are still waiting.) A true Strollercize mom would just turn around and let her butt do the talking. Trust me, when people see your big caboose coming at them, they'll get out of your way. Sure, your fellow shoppers might be upset that you have turned them into human sardines, but you have a life too. After all, there's shopping to be done.

LIFTING YOUR BABY

Lifting your baby is serious business. The majority of back injuries result from lifting heavy objects, and your baby certainly falls into that category. But when you do it the right way, lifting your baby can be a great muscle-building workout. In fact, the two basic methods for picking up a baby (see below) are based on moves from the gym. Whether you're lifting the baby, the television, or a bag of groceries, these three moves will serve you well.

How Not to Lift Your Baby. When left to their own devices, most people use a poor approximation of this move to lift heavy objects. They hang forward from their waists, reach out their arms, and lift the load with their back and arms rather than their legs (see photo below). The result is most certainly lower back pain and injury.

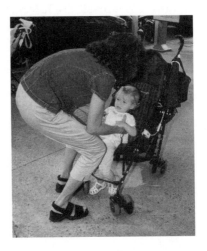

In the gym, they call this move the "dead lift." And it's developed such a bad reputation that it's been blacklisted by many trainers and national fitness organizations. Unfortunately, in the world outside the gym, the dead lift is a fact of life. There are times when bending forward is the only way to go. Besides, when done properly, the dead lift is not only safe, but it's a great way to stretch your legs and tone your rear end.

The Baby Lift

When lifting your baby in the *correct* dead lift position, follow the steps carefully to protect your back and tone your bod.

1. Stand facing your baby. Soften your knees, and hinge forward at your waist. Keep your chest lifted and your back flat. Your buns should be sticking out behind you, and your tummy should be tight. Think of yourself as a table. You're doing this right if you can balance a glass of water on your back.

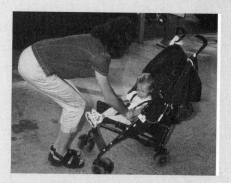

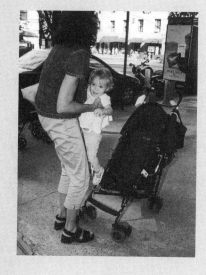

2. Now, grasp onto the baby under the armpits, with two fingers under the cranium if necessary. Bend your elbows, and use your biceps muscles to help your back.

3. Keep your chest lifted and your buttocks out as you lift the baby, your knees still soft, and return to standing. You should feel a nice stretch up the back of your legs, and a slight tension in your buttocks. If you feel any straining in your lower back, it means you're not doing this right. Check your form and try again. Remember to engage your abdominals.

The Squat

Here's another technique for lifting your baby, which is based on another traditional move from the gym: the squat. This move is great for moms with heavy babies or older toddlers and those who are already suffering from lower back pain. You'll draw most of your lifting strength from your leg muscles, so you'll be less likely to stress your lower back. But be warned—the squat can be a pretty intense workout for your buttocks and legs.

1. Start with your legs at least a shoulder-width apart. Bend your knees, and lower your buttocks out behind you and down to the floor. Your toes should be in line with your knees. Try to keep your heels on the ground. (This will be easier if you are wearing shoes.)

2. Grasp onto the baby, with your hands under her armpits, and bring her close to your body.

3. Keep your chest lifted as you slowly straighten your knees and return to standing.

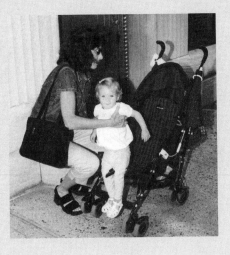

Remember, lifting is hard work. No matter how good your technique, you should still train your body to meet this daily challenge. Be sure to practice your Stroller Squats and Stroller Roll-Outs at least twice a week, along with the rest of your Bootie Camp routine (see Chapter 8). The stronger you are, the more likely you'll be to sail through this part of your daily obstacle course.

THE CAR

Unless you live in a big city as I do, where you can (and often must) walk everywhere, chances are that you and your baby will spend a lot of time in the car. Driving with a baby can be heavenly, because the motion and vibration usually lull her right to sleep. Getting the baby in and out of the car, however, can be a nightmare. You have to struggle with the squirming baby, those narrow doors, and of course, the dreaded car seat.

The Transfer

You probably transfer your baby in and out of the car at least a half-dozen times a day. Unfortunately, unless you own a very roomy car, and have an especially cooperative baby, it's never easy.

The trick to a safe transfer is to stay as close to the baby and to the car seat as possible. This way you will avoid all that unnecessary reaching, twisting, and turning.

1. Hold the baby close to your body, and climb inside the car—but don't sit down. Depending on your height, the size of the car, and the position of the car seat, step one or both legs inside the car.

2. To avoid unnecessary twisting and reaching, get as close to your child's safety seat as possible, and try to position your upper body directly in front of the seat. Transfer the baby into his seat.

3. After the baby is in the seat, step out of the car, stand erect, and take a few deep breaths. This will give your spine and muscles a chance to relax. When you feel ready, you can step back into the car (as described in steps 1 and 2) and strap the baby in.

Are You Ready for This?

Would you attempt a single-armed biceps curl with a 20-pound dumb-bell? Well, the average three-month-old baby/car seat combo can easily exceed twenty pounds. And the average parent is not equipped to handle it. That's why I tell all my clients that the best place for a car seat is in the car. Even if you are especially strong (read: a professional body builder), carrying a car seat is much harder on your body than lifting a dumbbell. Dumbbells can be gripped easily in one hand, held close to the body, and lifted while keeping your wrists and spine straight. It's nearly impossible, however, to maintain proper body alignment when carrying a car seat. The size and shape, let alone the awkward handle, contorts your body in ways that would make any physical therapist choke. And don't forget that after you've nearly killed yourself trying to lug that thing around, you still face the even more Herculean task of putting the seat (and the baby) into your car.

I realize that many of you will ignore my advice. After all, carrying your baby in the car seat is convenient, especially if you don't own a car. And there will probably be times when breaking your back seems like a minor inconvenience compared to waking the baby. If you must carry that car seat, never forget this one basic fact: You are not strong enough to carry your car seat with only one hand. If you're like most people, you'll wind up resting the car seat on your hip, while thrusting your weight to your opposite side to compensate for the load. The result: lower back strain, wrist pain, and severe shoulder injuries.

The best way to hold the car seat is with two hands (grasp either the handle or the base of the seat, whichever is more comfortable). Hold the seat in front of you, as close to your body as possible. Keep your back straight and your elbows bent at a 90-degree angle. For best results, avoid carrying your seat frequently or for extended periods of time.

DINNERTIME

Whether you breast- or bottle-feed your baby, feeding times are special times for bonding. But like almost everything else about mothering, it can also be a pain in the neck—literally. Bruised nipples, aching shoulders, and stiff necks seem to come with the territory. Here's how to protect your back when feeding your baby.

Breast-Feeding

The golden rule of breast-feeding is to bring the baby to the breast rather than the breast to the baby. Think about it: Your breasts are already hanging pretty low. Why pull them down any further? Besides, if you bring your breasts down to the baby, you'll be bringing your shoulders and chest with them. To minimize slouching, try to get the baby as high as possible. Raise your knees, use a few pillows, or buy a special breast-feeding cushion—whatever it takes to bring that baby up high and close to your breasts. If you're nursing on the couch or in a chair, try resting your feet on a footrest, an ottoman, or even the coffee table. This will help raise your lap up closer to your chest.

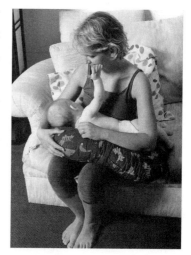

While it's important to find a comfortable place to feed the baby, don't let yourself get too comfortable. Flopping down on that big comfy couch or even the rocking chair can lead to less-than-perfect feeding posture. No matter where you settle down, remember to sit tall. Avoid rounding your spine and hunching your shoulders. Remember, you're a mom, not a rag doll.

Bottle-Feeding

I'll gladly stay out of the breast-versus-bottle debate. What I will tell you is that when it comes to posture, bottle-feeding moms don't have it any easier than their breast-feeding buddies. When giving your baby a bottle, you still need to be careful to maintain good sitting posture. That means that your spine is straight, your chest is lifted, and your shoulders are back and down.

To avoid a vicious case of "bottle elbow," be sure to keep the elbow of your feeding arm down and close to your body. Keep your wrist straight. I love those tilted bottles that you can hold at the proper feeding angle, without stressing your elbows and wrists. And don't forget to switch sides. Just as breast-feeding moms have to log in equal time on both breasts, bottle-feeders should remember to use both arms. That way the baby gets a change in view, and your arms and shoulders get a break.

THE END OF THE DAY

Congratulations, you've made it through another busy day. I have one last move that will strengthen your shoulders, while giving you a moment's peace: giving the baby to Daddy. At the end of the day, nothing is better than handing the baby over to your partner and jumping into a nice warm bubble bath.

Giving the Baby to Daddy

1. Hold the baby against your chest, with your hands around her chest and under her armpits, and your elbows bent and close to your body.

2. Slowly stretch out your arms to Daddy, and keep your torso erect and your knees soft. Hand the baby over to your partner. Keep your chest lifted and your tummy tight.

3. Blow the baby a kiss, and run!

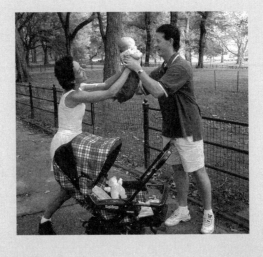

$$\cdots\cdots\cdots\cdots 11 \cdots\cdots\cdots\cdots$$

No More Excuses!

I'm too tired." "It's raining." "I don't have time" Believe me, I've heard all the excuses for not exercising. And I understand—it's hard enough to start a new exercise program even when you don't have a new baby in your life. Now that you're a mom, it may seem darn near impossible. But you can find a place in your new life for fitness. From making the time to braving the elements, this chapter addresses all of the common excuses and obstacles to starting a postpartum exercise program. At the end of this chapter, I'll give you some tips for sticking with your Strollercize program for years to come.

MY BABY WON'T SIT IN THE STROLLER

One of the first things moms ask when they call to sign up for Strollercize classes is "What if my baby won't sit in the stroller?" I understand their concern, but the truth is that most babies love to Strollercize. Few babies can resist the motion of the stroller and the stimulating scenery, not to mention the joy of watching Mom work up a sweat.

Of course, some babies don't like strollers as a rule, and any baby can have a bad day. If your baby doesn't like the stroller on your first day out, don't give up. In my experience, it usually takes about three tries before the baby is Strollercized. If after a few outings you're still having trouble, try changing your route or working out at a different time of the day. And always remember to feed the baby before you stroll. If all else fails, you can try planning your workouts during your baby's regular nap time. The trick is to keep trying until you find a routine that works. Trust me, if exercise is really important to you, your baby will learn to compromise.

THE WEATHER IS TERRIBLE

I know the story: It's pouring rain or freezing cold, and there's no way you're leaving the house. But the fact is that there are no perfect climates, and even if you live in a sunny area, the weather will sooner or later threaten to get in the way of your workout. Here in New York City, Strollercize classes are packed year-round, rain or shine. If we're not afraid of a little bad weather, why should you be? A bit of fresh air in those cold winter months will do wonders for your spirits, and if you're properly equipped, a few drops of rain never drowned anyone's spirit.

Of course, you may have to take some extra precautions. In the dog days of summer, an early morning or evening workout is best. Wear light clothes, and dress the baby in a onesie or even just a diaper. Stay out of direct sunlight, and don't forget the sunglasses and sunblock. (Most sunblocks are only appropriate for babies six months and older; check with your doctor.) You may also want to invest in a sunshade for the stroller (e.g., an umbrella or a Strollercize Peek-a-Boo cover). In the dead of winter, layering your clothes is essential. Go for fabrics that are especially designed for winter workouts, and don't forget the hat and gloves. To avoid catching a chill, cover up before you start to cool down. And always change out of your wet clothes as soon as possible. Keep in mind that while you're huffing and puffing, the baby is sitting still. She'll need to stay bundled, even if you're starting to feel warm.

No matter what the weather report says, always pack rain gear—just in case. Those plastic shields (never use ordinary plastic trash bags) are great not only for keeping the baby dry but for beating the wind-chill factor on blustery days. And since a light sprinkle can turn into a heavy downpour with little warning, it's a good idea to work out where there is shelter nearby. Take care on wet pavement, which can get slippery, and if it's hazy or foggy, be sure to stay well out of the way of automobile traffic and bicyclists.

Some weather conditions really aren't worth braving. Never Strollercize on an icy road or sidewalk. Never go out when there is a thunderstorm, hurricane, or tornado. And if the weatherman says it's too hot or too cold for small children, you and the baby should stay indoors. If you do find yourself stuck inside on a miserable day, don't give up. You can always head to the mall or do some of the moves in your living room. The exercises in Chapter 5 work just as well indoors as out.

I'M TOO TIRED

I know you're tired. Even if your new baby is sleeping "through the night," that usually means you'll be up at four A.M. But here's a shocker: Working out will give you more energy! I know it's hard to think about going for a stroll when you're too tired to walk to the bathroom. But it really does help. How else do you think, as a single mother of three, I manage to run my own business? Honestly, I'd never have the energy to get through my day if I didn't work out.

Of course, it's hard to get motivated to exercise on four hours of sleep. That's why you should try to get as much rest as possible, and to save what little energy you have for the important things, like caring for the baby and Strollercizing. Everyone will tell you to sleep when the baby sleeps, but truthfully this never worked for me. By the time I managed to clear my head and settle down in bed, the baby would wake up and be ready to go. Besides, I wanted to catch up on life when the baby slept. Sometimes that meant sitting on the sofa reading a magazine. Other times I just wound up staring at the wall. And if by some stroke of luck, my head fell back on the sofa and I got a quick nap, then that was great, too.

Those restful catnaps really come in handy when a longer nap is out of the question. Other forms of the catnap include watching an old movie, organizing a list of things to do, or just meditating. The trick is to choose activities that you find restful and refreshing. Remember, rest helps you care for your new baby, maintain a strong milk supply, and recover from pregnancy and birth.

One more thing. You may find that you have more energy to exercise in the morning. Studies show that people who work out early in the day are more likely to stick with their program. It makes sense. If you wait until the end of the day, you may be too tired to get off the couch, let alone go for a stroll.

I'M TOO FAT

Here's the paradox: To lose the weight, you have to work out. But if you're like many new moms, you may feel much too fat to exercise. I know how you feel. When I headed back to work after the birth of my third child, Romeu, nobody could believe I was the instructor. With my bulging belly and well-padded hips, I didn't exactly look like the model of fitness. But that didn't stop me, and it shouldn't stop you! The truth is that exercise will help you feel better about your body.

Before you can improve your figure, you'll have to improve your self-image. Here are some tips for feeling good about yourself—and your (bigger) bod.

Change Your Wardrobe! Even if you're not wearing the size you'd like to be, get rid of the pregnancy clothes and buy a few new outfits. Choose comfortable activewear that will make you feel energized. Treat yourself to some lacy underwear and a sexy bra. Yes, your condition is temporary. But you still deserve to feel pretty, sexy, and free.

Give Yourself a "Face-lift"! Wash your face with your favorite cleanser, and smooth on a luxurious moisturizer. If you like perfume, spray on your best scent, and let the aroma lift your mood. Even if you don't normally wear makeup, a little lip gloss, blush, and mascara can make you feel human again. If you did this routine before the baby arrived and you've stopped, get back in the habit! It's the little things that will make you feel like your old self.

Eat Right! Unfortunately, Mom's healthy food habits usually drop off faster than the body fat. You can't find the time to eat a sensible meal, so you eat whatever you can get your hands on. But those junk foods can leave you feeling sluggish, bloated, and guilty. Instead, choose foods that will nourish you both physically and mentally. The following tips should help:

- Always eat a big breakfast. Never skip this meal.
- Eat foods for fuel, not just for flavor.
- Never eat standing up, especially in front of the refrigerator.
- Never finish everything on your plate.
- Eat colorfully (i.e., lots of whole grains, fruits, and vegetables).
- Never skip meals.
- Dangerous food hours are 2 to 4 P.M. and after 8:30 P.M.—be careful!
- Do not eat a big meal after 7:30 at night!
- Always have a healthy snack on hand.
- Drink plenty of water (at least 8 cups a day). It's easy to confuse thirst and hunger.
- Dilute your favorite juice with equal parts of water, to satisfy your taste buds without adding too many extra calories.
- Eat one hour before Strollercizing.
- Fast foods are a sure way to find fat on your body!

Healthy eating is hard work, but it's worth the effort. Not only will you lose those last few (or not so few) pounds, but you'll feel better about your body if you know you're putting the right stuff into it.

I CAN'T FIND THE TIME

You've got to feed the baby, change the baby, dress the baby, remove spit-up stains from the baby and from the couch, dress the baby again, feed the baby again, change the baby again. You still need to clean the house, take a shower, call the office, cook dinner, return ten phone calls, and read the mail. Exercise now? You've got to be kidding.

Okay, don't panic. You may think that you have no time. But this is the wrong way to think. If you don't *have* the time, you'll have to *make* it. Prioritize. Write a list of all the things you really need to do, and put Strollercize at the top. Set the schedule. And don't be afraid to say no to anything that's not absolutely necessary. It's okay to leave the beds unmade and a few dust bunnies under the sofa. Your first priority is to take care of yourself and the baby. Everything else will fall into place . . . eventually.

One great way to take control of your time is to make a daily itinerary. Write a list of everything that needs to be done—errands, phone calls, thank-you notes, Strollercize—and then fit each one into your time chart. Be clear about which activities are absolutely essential, and which ones can wait for another day. Once you get in the habit, you'll see how easy it is to fit a little exercise into your busy day. Here's a sample:

MORNING

6:00 A.M.

Wake up and prepare yourself for the day. If the baby is sleeping, jump in the shower and try to shave both legs! Fix breakfast and some healthy snacks for later in the day.

7:00 A.M.

The baby is up! It's time to play Mom. Feed him, dress him, bathe him—whatever your morning ritual involves. If you work outside of the home, this might be your only chance to Strollercize. If you don't have time now, gather up your workout gear so you'll be ready to go when you get home from work.

8:00 A.M.

Baby takes her morning nap. This could be a catnap moment for Mom. If you can't settle down, make a list of the day's to-do activities. This is also the time to get yourself ready to go out.

9:30 A.M.

The baby is awake, and you should be ready to leave the house. This is a good time for grocery shopping because the stores are not busy and you are fresh. (If you wait until later, you'll be tired, hungry, and more likely to buy out the store.) If you opt to stay home, take this time to conquer some of those household chores. How is the laundry situation? Do the plants need watering? Your energy level is still high (relatively speaking), so use it well.

11:00 A.M.

This is the perfect time to Strollercize. The day's still young, and you're feeling in top form (or close enough). Grab your gear, and get moving!

AFTERNOON

12:30 P.M.

Lunchtime. How about going out to a restaurant with a fellow mother?

2:00 p.m.

The baby's napping again, or he may want to play. Take a catnap if you can, do your Strollercize Waist Away routine (see Chapter 5), or get a head start on preparing dinner. This is a good time to get things done because you are not completely exhausted yet.

4:00 P.M.

If you did not work out in the morning, this is another good time to Strollercize. You may be feeling the end-of-the-day blahs, and exercise can give you a second wind. If you already worked out, then enjoy this quiet time to watch *Oprah,* catch up on your thank-you notes, or start up your own home business, like me!

EVENING

5:00 P.M.

Attention, working mothers: Here's another opportunity to Strollercize. Change into your workout gear as soon as you come home. Then get out of the house before you start to feel too comfortable on that couch.

7:00 P.M.

Fix dinner. Eat dinner. Feed the baby. Especially for working mothers, this is bound to be the most difficult time of the day. Need to let off some steam? Go for a stroll, or just chill on the front porch and get some air.

8:00 P.M.

Bathe the baby. Feed the baby. And try to get her settled down for the night. You deserve some time for yourself—especially if you've been home all day with the baby. If possible, hang up your "off duty" sign and have Dad do the honors.

9:00 P.M.

Relax! Call a friend, take a bubble bath, and get ready to take care of the biggest baby—your husband—in the house. He needs the most changing, cuddling—and should I say breast-feeding? Your marriage needs this nurturing time. Cuddle up and talk.

LATE NIGHT AND THE WEE, WEE HOURS

10:15 P.M.

Put on a new nightgown, and catch up on your reading. Try to go to bed early, because you may be up in a few hours.

2:00 A.M.

Feed or check on the baby. Get a bowl of cereal or fruit to nourish yourself, especially if you are breast-feeding.

4:00 A.M.

You may need to get up again, especially if your baby is younger than six months. Try the early morning weird shows for entertainment, or watch the weather forecast to predict your day's outings. The sun may be rising soon.

6:00 A.M.

Get up, Mom—here we go again. Exercise will give you the energy you need to make it through the wee, wee hours.

Keep in mind that this schedule is not designed for a working mom or even a mom like me with three children. Being raised in the port of Seattle helped me to be the captain of a life that is like the *Titanic*. I am always on the verge of sinking. For all the moms out there, you have plenty of lifeboats (friends and family). Use them. Moms are survivors.

STICK WITH IT!

Getting back in shape after having a baby is hard work. It takes time, effort, and a lot of patience. If you're not seeing the results that you hoped for—and even if you are—it may be difficult to stick with your program. All of those things that made it difficult to start exercising in the first place will still be around long after you've established a regular exercise routine. You'll never have enough time. The weather won't always be perfect. And there will always be days when getting off the couch seems as daunting as climbing Mount Everest. The good news is that once you've learned to make fitness a part of your life, you probably won't be able to live without it.

Of course, making exercise a part of your life is easier said than done. So many people start exercise programs only to abandon them days, weeks, or months later. In my experience, it takes about three months to get into the rhythm of a regular exercise program and another six months for your workouts to become an essential part of your life. In the meantime, the following tips should help you stay motivated:

Be Consistent. To get in the habit of exercising, consistency is key. If you skip a few weeks (or even a few workouts), it will be harder to get back to your program. Try to set aside a regular time each week for your workout (the way you do for doctors' appointments or play dates). And when the time comes, force yourself to go, even if you don't feel like it. Prepare yourself ahead of time by changing into your workout clothes and packing your stroller (that's half the battle). And keep the "appointment," no matter how lazy you feel.

Sometimes the hardest part of a workout is getting started. Whether you're too tired or too busy or just not in the mood, there will be times when you're tempted to skip your routine. Don't do it! Force yourself to exercise, even if you aim for only five or ten minutes. Chances are that once you get moving, you won't want to stop.

Don't Do It Alone. Being a mother can be isolating. But exercise doesn't have to be. A big part of the New York City Strollercize classes is that a group of moms get together to support each other's efforts. If a mom's feeling tired or her baby is fussing, we all rally around her and give her the support and encouragement she needs to keep going. If you can't find a Strollercize class in your area (don't worry, there's one coming soon), you can get some of the same benefits by asking your spouse or another mom to be your Strollercize partner. Find someone with similar experiences and similar goals. That way you can shoot the breeze while helping each other stay focused and fit.

Focus on the Positive. If the pounds aren't dropping as fast as you'd like them to, or if your tummy is still looking flabby, you may be tempted to give up and go back to that couch. Bad idea! Reevaluate your diet, step up your exercise intensity, and stick with it. Remember, it took you nine months to put on the weight, and it can easily take a year to lose it. But you'll be reaping the benefits of exercising long before you lose your last pound.

Don't Forget to Have Fun! Your workouts should be fun, not stressful. While you're Strollercizing, focus on how good you feel, not on how many pounds you're losing or the number of hours you spend working out. The early days of motherhood pass very quickly. If you're caught up in trying to get back to normal too quickly, you may miss some of what makes this time so special.

Despite your best efforts, you may still fall off the exercise wagon. Don't beat yourself up. Just get moving again! After all, if you've spent years being sedentary, it may be hard to change those ways overnight. The trick is to keep trying, until you discover what works for you. You can do it, Mom!

Beyond Strollercize

Someday your child will grow out of the stroller. Your baby will grow up and go to school, and you may even go back to the gym. Times will change, and you'll change along with them.

I hope Strollercize has taught you to make the commitment to fitness. Moms need to be strong and fit and to spend as much time with their children as possible. Your children will follow in your footsteps, your strides, and your rolls. If you show them the way of a healthy lifestyle, you'll give them the gift of fitness as well.

It's been ten years since I first started Strollercizing, and I have had the pleasure of sharing this program with thousands of new moms. As I stroll in Central Park with my third and last child, Romeu, age 3, Tatiana, age 10, Rollerblades along, and Lorenzo, at 8, soars ahead on his bicycle. The wheels of my life will keep turning. Someday I'll be pushing my grandchild in a stroller, and pulling up the rear of a class of new moms—but right behind me will be a whole bunch of grandmas! May the benefits of Strollercize carry you through your parenting years and beyond.

Resources

STROLLERCIZE® offers:

- 100 indoor and outdoor classes in Manhattan
- Fitness accessories for Mom
- Video workouts for Mom and Dad
- Babyweight™ toning tools
- Expansion programs
- Stroller shopping advice

Surf the Web while breast feeding; it's fun! Here are some great Web sites to check out:

BabyGap.com

Urbanbaby.com

FitPregnancy.com

Babystyle.com

LifeServ.com

AmericanBaby.com

Parentsplace.com

BabyCenter.com

Mom.com

Please contact us for our updated resource list:

Strollercize Incorporated
New York, New York
www.strollercize.com
Phone: 1–800–Y-STROLL
E-mail: ystroll@strollercize.com

Credits

The following Strollercize moms and their children are featured in this book. I'd like to offer my gratitude for their time and enthusiasm.

- Kimberly Ajavanada with Reilly Ajavanada (born 5/17/99)
- Denise Brecher with Jamie Lerner-Brecher (born 4/5/95) and Matthew Lerner-Brecher (born 3/10/98)
- Claudia Costa-Pinto with Tomas Greenberg (born 7/30/99)
- Paul Campbell with Bryan (born 4/25/00)
- Jill Dachman with Benjamin Dachman (born 10/29/99)
- Laura Dougherty with Claudia Dougherty (born 9/29/98)
- Linda Humphrey with Jack Humphrey (born 5/17/99)
- Margaret Kaufer with Liam Bishop Kaufer (born 1/26/98) and Hannah Lee Kaufer (born 10/8/99)
- Nancy Levine with A.J. (born 4/28/98) and Dylan (born 9/9/99)
- Donna Rodolitz with Jason Rodolitz (born 10/21/99)
- Claudine Rosenthal with Alexis Rosenthal (born 12/8/99)
- Sharon Sharofsky-Mack with Rebecca Mack (born 7/26/94) and Jonathan Mack (born 3/6/99)
- Victoria Shaw with Camille Shaw-Faucheux (born 4/18/97) and Julian Shaw-Faucheux (born 9/26/99)
- Melissa Shildkraut with Madeline (born 6/10/96)
- Margaret Smith with Connor Michael Smith (born 12/16/99)
- Shirra Stone with Emmett Stone (born 8/23/99) and Fiona Stone (born 3/19/96)
- Terry Voltaggio with Liliana Voltaggio (born 10/14/99)
- Mary Woods with Sara McCloskey (born 6/2/99)
- And Elizabeth Trindade with Tatiana (born 2/11/90) Lorenzo (born 6/2/92) and Romeu (born 5/2/97)

All photographs were taken by Arthur Julian of Style Studios and Gill King of Gill King Photography.

Index

physical fitness (*cont.*)
    components of, 30–31
    described, 29–30
    weight control and, 30, 31, 172–73
    See also exercise
postpartum depression, 20, 21
posture, 52–57, 144
prams, 40–41
push-ups, 132, 134

quadriceps, 60, 101, 108

realistic goals, setting, 31–32
relaxin (hormone), 23, 24
RICE system for injuries, 59
running, 35, 108

safety
    exercise, 63–65
    stroller, 43–44
sex life, 21
shins, 59, 91
shin splits, 24–25, 59
shoulders
    exercises for, 103, 132, 135, 136
    muscles, 61
    posture and, 55
    strain, 25–26
    stretch, 144
    warmup exercise, 86–87
sleep deprivation, 20
social life, 20
sports bra, 47
squats, 112, 164
stiff neck, 26
stress incontinence, 23, 63, 67
stretching, 141–49
strollers
    curbs and, 155–56

doorway maneuvering, 154–55
elevators and, 161
folding, 156–57
lifting, 158–59
safety, 43–44
selection tips, 43–45
stairs and, 159–60
test driving, 45–46
types of, 39–43
strolling. *See* aerobic exercise; walking

target heart-rate zone, 95
tennis elbow, 26, 61
thighs
    exercises for, 101, 102, 112, 116,
      119
    muscles in, 60–61
    warmup exercises, 88, 89, 90
    See also hamstrings; quadriceps
three-wheeler strollers, 42
travel systems, 42

umbrella strollers, 41

waistline. *See* abdomen/abdominals
walking
    hills, 108
    suggested pace, 96, 107
    vs. driving, 33
warmup exercises, 85–93, 110
warning signs, 35
Washington, Yakima, 42
water, 50
weight control, 30, 31, 172–73
wrists, 61
    exercises for, 138
    pain, 26, 166
    posture and, 55–56

About the Authors

ELIZABETH TRINDADE is the founder of Strollercize®, which conducts more than one hundred classes a month in New York City and has recently licensed instructors from Seattle to Boston. VICTORIA SHAW has taught classes in child development at Princeton and Columbia Universities. Both authors live in New York.